The Tao of K-drama

NARRATIVE MEDICINE SERIES

Series Editors
Maura Spiegel, Craig Irvine, Rita Charon, *Columbia University*

Published in the Series

THE TAO OF K-DRAMA
Wise Narratives for a Troubled World
Mindy Thompson Fullilove, MD

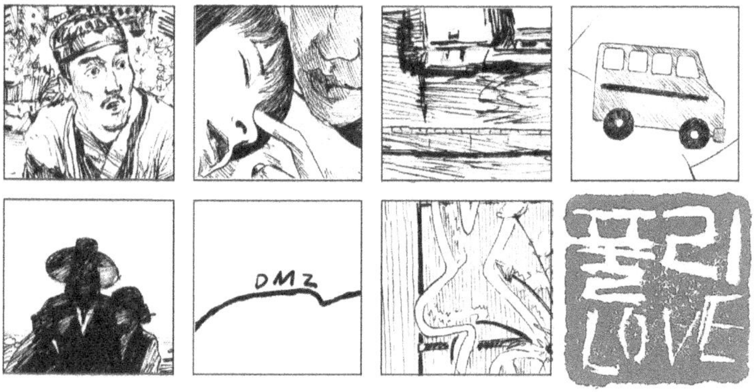

The Tao of K-drama

Wise Narratives for a Troubled World

MINDY THOMPSON FULLILOVE, MD

OXFORD
UNIVERSITY PRESS

OXFORD
UNIVERSITY PRESS

Oxford University Press is a department of the University of Oxford. It furthers the University's objective of excellence in research, scholarship, and education by publishing worldwide. Oxford is a registered trade mark of Oxford University Press in the UK and in certain other countries.

Published in the United States of America by Oxford University Press
546 Fifth Avenue, New York, NY 10036, United States of America.

CIP data is on file at the Library of Congress

ISBN 978-0-19-784697-1

DOI: 10.1093/med/9780197846971.001.0001

Printed by Integrated Books International, United States of America

The manufacturer's authorized representative in the EU for product safety is Oxford University Press España S.A. of Parque Empresarial San Fernando de Henares, Avenida de Castilla, 2 – 28830 Madrid (www.oup.es/en or product.safety@oup.com). OUP España S.A. also acts as importer into Spain of products made by the manufacturer.

MIX
Paper
FSC FSC® C183721

For my children, Bobby, Kenny, Dina, and Molly
Shelter in the Storm

“72-year-old woman 15,000 miles from home”

because in COVID time a tv show comforted me
I am smelling the painter’s lilacs instead of my own
watching the sunset behind Daughter-in-Law Rock
and appreciating paintings of Hell

the first painting depicts a man in a gas mask holding
his heart
the second a starving dog with his head stuck in a jar
the third a Buddha’s young face with a yellow ribbon
to remind us of the ferry disaster

on the train back to Seoul a child peeks at me with curiosity
so her mother encourages her to make friends—
she cautiously hands me a mint and later says
“anyong” and waves a sleepy goodbye

home is not 15,000 miles away, as my granddaughter said,
but 6,900, and my knee is feeling fine today.

Mindy Fullilove

Contents

Figures and Tables

Figures

Tables

Series Editors' Foreword

Maura Spiegel, Craig Irvine, Rita Charon

This volume inaugurates a new book series devoted to narrative medicine. Narrative medicine draws on skills and habits of attention from the humanities and the arts to engage questions of health, illness, and care, bringing perspectives from fields such as phenomenology, literary criticism, visual studies, and psychoanalysis into conversation with clinical practice. Attentiveness to narrative offers ways of understanding the embodied experience of illness that extend beyond instrumental intervention and remain responsive to the complexities of lived experience. As the field has evolved, it has continued to expand its objects of study, its methods, and its cultural reach.

Our aspiration for this series is to widen the aperture of narrative medicine still further: to welcome new voices, methods, and objects of study; to remain attentive to the ways narrative knowledge circulates beyond traditional clinical or academic settings; and to invite fresh approaches to understanding suffering, repair, and connection. The books to come engage the field's established commitments while also drawing insight from work that crosses disciplines, challenges assumptions, and takes shape in diverse cultural and global contexts.

It is fitting that the series begins with ***The Tao of K-Drama: Wise Narratives for a Troubled World***. Drawing on four decades of work as a social psychiatrist studying epidemics of suffering in poor and marginalized communities, Mindy Fullilove turns her attention to Korean television drama as a narrative form deeply attuned to upheaval, trauma, and the struggle to reconnect in the face of despair. As she writes, when she first encountered K-drama, she recognized that its writers were grappling with the same human crises that have shaped her own work. We offer this book as our beginning.

Foreword

Jae Shin 신재윤

Why would a social psychiatrist who studies cities write about K-drama? Dr. Mindy Fullilove has spent years tracing ruptures in urban environments, studying how they shape cities, unsettle communities, and demand restoration. During the COVID-19 pandemic, she started watching K-dramas. The idea of someone steeped in academic work and deeply engaged in structural thinking binge-watching melodramas was both surprising and, to me, perfectly fitting. Though the study of what shapes the urban landscape and the study of K-drama inhabit vastly different worlds, in both, Dr. Fullilove parses how people come together, form coalitions, and navigate the work of rebuilding what has been broken.

As a Korean American who grew up watching K-dramas, I bonded with her over the juicy aesthetics and tropes of the genre: lavish dinner tables covered in *banchan* (반찬, side dishes), over-the-top love triangles or squares, family dramas among *chaebol* (재벌, large, family-controlled business conglomerates), and the satisfying narratives of *gwon-seon-jing-ak* (권선징악, poetic justice). In typical Dr. Fullilove fashion, she soon went deeper—taking intensive Korean language lessons, closely attending to linguistic patterns that reflect cultural ways of relating. When she talked to me about the sense of connection and mutuality embodied in the Korean word *oori* (우리, we or us), it made sense, given her focus on networks of belonging, that she would be drawn to a word so deeply rooted in relational ways of being.

I came to know Dr. Fullilove's work through *Root Shock: How Tearing Up City Neighborhoods Hurts America and What We Can*

Do About It, her 2004 book on the psychological and social impacts of displacement, which includes stories from three American cities: Newark, New Jersey; Pittsburgh, Pennsylvania; and Roanoke, Virginia. As a graduate student of architecture working on my thesis project, I studied the legacy of urban renewal in Newark, where aggressive government takings of land through eminent domain had produced lasting damage. Five decades later, that damage was still visible in monolithic urban blocks of university and hospital campuses, consolidated vacant lots, and the highways and corridors that cut through them. Dr. Fullilove's unpacking of how "the distinction between social and physical aspects of the environment is an arbitrary one" grounded my project. It shaped my argument that the public benefits promised in exchange for destroying neighborhoods—social services, community programming, institutional giving—must be made legible not only through social programs but also through physical improvements, and vice versa.

Dr. Fullilove's work guides my approach to urban design and planning and my search for ways to make clear links between physically making a place—its parks, houses, sidewalks, bike racks—and the social and political forces among which it exists. Her account of urban renewal's "social costs of displacement" in a city where authorities intended "to clear nearly half the land . . . and displace one in seven residents" is a reminder of the power structures that shape the city and how hierarchies of power and class are reflected in the material details of the built environment.

Dr. Fullilove's work on place politics—*Root Shock* and her two subsequent books, *Urban Alchemy: Restoring Joy in America's Sorted-Out Cities* (2013) and *Main Street: How a City's Heart Connects Us All* (2020)—offers much for urban design and planning practitioners interested in the relationship between the physical and the social life of a city. Whereas the training of architects and designers often foregrounds reading the city through form and materiality, her work points toward pedagogy that makes legible a city marked by enduring struggles over the built environment and the power structures that shape it. In her framing, social and structural disconnection reinforce one another in a feedback loop: "The divided city is a subjugated city." Her work points designers toward practices rooted in concrete experience and collective action. It helps us understand how meaning operates in the environment: how urban design can help and harm public health, and how community organizing and popular education can serve as forms of recovery. She often unpacks this working of collectivity through the concept of the "mazeway," showing how a place is made meaningful through collective experience.

The mazeway, a term developed by Anthony F. C. Wallace, is not simply the physical layout and character of a location; it describes a complex interplay of meaning and material, where the physical environment is an important ingredient in how people make sense of their lives and recognize their place in the world. In *Root Shock* and beyond, Dr. Fullilove describes how federal urban renewal programs ruptured and destroyed mazeways, leading to social group paralysis. Understood positively, the design and affordances of human environments explain themselves to us, connect us to places, and transmit messages about human dignity, worth, and agency.

This "sum of the lifeways in a community," the mazeway, resonates with *oori*, the word Dr. Fullilove noted as distinctive. It means "we" or "us" in Korean, but unlike in English—where "we" usually defines a group in opposition to others—it reflects a relational worldview. It's not about drawing a boundary; it's about embeddedness. It shows up everywhere in daily speech: "우리 집" (*oori jip*, our house), even if you live alone; "우리 언니" (*oori unni*, our sister), even when referring to your only sibling; "우리 남편" (*oori nampyun*, our husband), in a monogamous relationship!

In these everyday expressions, *oori* doesn't mean literal shared ownership; it signals relationship. When Koreans say "우리 동네" (*oori dongnae*, our neighborhood) or "우리 나라" (*oori nara*, our country) to mean "my neighborhood" or "my country," it lands differently than it would for an English speaker using those same words. The emphasis is less on possession and more on mutuality, situating the self within the collective. This is where Dr. Fullilove's mazeways and the Korean grammar of *oori* converge; both describe systems of connection that shape how we navigate the world, not alone but in relation.

Oori signals not a boundary between groups but a relational embeddedness—a state of belonging. What Dr. Fullilove surfaces—through her earlier descriptions of mazeways and her attention to *oori* in *The Tao of K-Drama: Wise Narratives for a Troubled World*—is that it isn't merely a cultural artifact or a linguistic feature; rather, it's a sociopolitical practice. Like the notion of *gongdongche* (공동체, collectivity), *oori* helps us understand how people hold one another through place, story, and shared purpose.

Because of this, when I first heard about Dr. Fullilove's writing on Korean dramas, I knew it wouldn't be an exercise in cultural appreciation that explores aesthetics, global reception, or representational politics. Rather, as in all her work, it would be an interdisciplinary unpacking of her theory of change, grounded in a community shaped by shared lifeways and place politics and, this time, joyfully conveyed through her narrative analysis of these fabulous stories.

In her writing on cities, Dr. Fullilove often turns to the image of a transect, a method of sampling used in ecology and field biology, a linear slice along which species and conditions are recorded, and a concept adapted by design fields like landscape architecture, urban design, and planning to describe variation across an urban gradient. A transect moves through varied neighborhoods and terrains, cutting across urban, suburban, and infrastructural spaces. Dr. Fullilove uses it as a method for reading the city in context, attending to shifts in density, land use, and social fabric. Described as "a form of horizontal archaeology," it is also a pedagogical journey. Walking the transect means encountering the city's contradictions through its ruptures and repairs, its missteps and moments of collective imagination. In this book I see her extending the use of that linear figure into the realm of narrative, offering the "arc of restoration" as a kind of relational transect. The full duration of a K-drama—eight, sixteen, or sometimes twenty episodes—becomes the unit through which repair is stretched, tested, and made visible. We learn what it looks like to stay in relationship through disorientation, conflict, and recovery.

This is an extension of Dr. Fullilove's longstanding practice of bringing disciplines together: psychiatry, urban planning, public health, design, and popular education. She has stayed close to the real-world consequences of practice, whether through her work cofounding the University of Orange, a people's free university in Orange, New Jersey, or serving as public director on the board of directors of the American Institute of Architects. Her work is generous to multiple modes of knowledge, while demanding rigor and long-term commitment from practitioners.

Because her work engages multiple disciplines, it invites further interdisciplinary interpretation and application. Practitioners in many fields might draw from her work to shape methods that reflect their own contexts. The possibilities for creative invention are vast, especially for practitioners forging many new paths for *oori*. In my case, it has led to a method used in the neighborhood planning or design process we undertake. We begin by forming an organizational steering committee made up of representatives from civic units: faith institutions, tenant associations, block clubs, nonprofits—people who have long done the work of holding neighborhoods together. These aren't individual volunteers with good intentions; they represent relationships and visions, efforts and networks that have been honed through the hard and patient work of community organizing. When these groups advise and lead a planning process from beginning to end, neighborhood planning cannot be reduced to a checklist of physical improvements or policy fixes. Instead, it becomes a collaborative opportunity: a space to negotiate across existing efforts, to recognize patterns of overlap, and to chart a shared path forward.

The durability of *oori* is often tested in K-dramas, as Dr. Fullilove points out in this book, and similarly, coalitions in real life are fragile. We all work within the precarious conditions of democracy, where conflicts abound, resources are uneven, and shared interests are constantly recalculated. And yet, it is that work of coalition building in finding shared ground that forms the civic unit capable of holding together our mazeways, our shared experience of living in cities.

That narrative of coalition, central to the structure of many K-dramas, where an *oori* forms and travels together through the narrative arc, isn't just literary. It's instructional. It offers those of us engaged in community work a powerful metaphor and method: to build durable *oori*, not by asserting unity, but by practicing shared navigation through complexity.

That's why this book is for anyone who loves a good television drama, and for those who are also invested in building their own theory of change within and beyond their disciplinary limit. It's for those drawn to the patient, careful work of narrativizing a journey and for those skeptical of letting first impressions, like the surface form or material of a city, define what is legible. Constructing a theory of change requires stories: stories rooted in mazeways, built up over time, and situated in real environments. Whether it's about cities or K-dramas, Dr. Fullilove's writing invites us to pay attention, to understand what shapes our collectivity through the networks of people, places, and struggles we endure.

Acknowledgments

Writing about K-drama has been an extraordinary privilege and pleasure. I am grateful, first and foremost, to all the artists who have created such a treasury of vivid stories. I was "home alone" during the COVID shelter in place when I discovered K-drama. It lifted my spirits, comforted my soul, and provided me with community. And clearly, given the genre's worldwide popularity, the artists know how to use the specific to convey the universal to their global audience.

Many, many people have supported me and made it possible to learn about dramas in a new language and from a culture not my own. I am indebted to them all. Michael Lally, Leo Anderson, and Derek Park hold a special place in this process because their unbounded enthusiasm provided both support and incentive. Professor Kyla Park, who has taught me the Korean language, early on announced that she was "taking responsibility" for me, in the Korean sense, and that has made all the difference. Maura Speigel and Craig Irvine identified that my book fit in the genre of narrative medicine and proposed it to Oxford University Press. The support and affirmation of their colleague Rita Charon, who is a founder of the discipline of narrative medicine, is one of the great honors of my life. Vivian Heller and Robert Fullilove have read many versions of the manuscript and been unflagging in their enthusiasm and on point with excellent advice. Susan Hasho and Robert Sember served as developmental editors and helped me bring my ideas into a felicitous whole.

Many friends and colleagues in the US have shared my love of K-drama and helped me deepen my understanding. Jae Shin was the first of many friends I contacted to share my original astonishment, and it is fitting that her foreword brings our conversation full circle. Hilda Hutcherson, Janis Blumgart, Irene Yen, Karen Love, and Hali Breindel participated in a stimulating series of conversations about K-drama. Laura Van Vleet, Liam Van Vleet, Sarah Kirshen, Ayako Maruyama, and Molly Kaufman were members of TV Club, and we worked together to write a paper on "Crash Landing on You" (CLOY). Professor Hope Elizabeth May introduced me to her world of Memory Parlors, which helped connect pieces of the story of Korea to that of the United States. Sarah Howe, who had lived in Korea for five years, shared stories, insights, and descriptions of K-drama horror shows, a subgenre I do not follow but she does.

I taught "Situation Analysis Through the Lens of K-Drama" for two wonderful semesters at The New School, and the students produced collections of essays that have helped me dig deep into K-drama. Each class named the situation depicted in the show, and I have used those names as chapter titles. My undergraduate class on Root Shock worked closely with me through a semester that was challenged by war and climate change yet allowed us to affirm the validity of what I learned from K-drama.

During my visit to the Republic of Korea, I was welcomed by many people, first and foremost by Drs. Howard Waitzkin and Mira Lee, who kindly connected me to their network of public health leaders. Dr. Lee Bora[1] and her family oriented me to the history and current moment in South Korea. When I tripped, she referred me to the amazing Dr. Kim Yi-jong, who got me back on my feet. And when I got COVID at the end of my visit, she took me to see a pulmonologist and provided me with medicines for each and every one of my symptoms. Dr. Kong Jeong-ok and her husband, Joe DiGangi, shared their love of K-drama and insights into the role of stories in Korean culture. Howard and Mira introduced me to their neighbor, the remarkable artist Byun Jeong Dae-seob, and we spent a miraculous time in his garden. Byun Jeong Dae-seob gave permission to use his remarkable painting, *Red Mirror*, made in remembrance of the 2014 Sewol Ferry disaster. As 250 of the 304 people who died were high school students, the painting depicts the face of a youth, while the yellow signifies the ribbons worn in protest of the mismanagement of the tragedy. He also connected me to Professor Eunju Hwang, who offered innumerable kinds of help, including showing me "secrets of Seoul" and making sure I had delicious food while in quarantine with COVID.

Architect EJ Lee, with help from her sister, introduced me to K-drama writer Kim Won-seok and translated for us during a lovely luncheon. She also helped me organize a temple stay at Tongdosa. I am grateful to the monks and temple volunteers who cared for me while I was there. I met artist Lee Kyungho at Tongdosa and later got to spend an enthralling afternoon at his studio in Seoul. I had the honor of presenting several lectures during my visit, and I am grateful to all the organizations that hosted me. I am particularly grateful to Dr. Changhyun Jang, who taught me that "hegemonic mimicry" is a real thing.

Family and friends have offered many kinds of help throughout the course of this project. Molly Rose Kaufman, Douglas Farrand, Marisela Gomez, Véronique Héon-Klin, Lily Johnson, Gahlia Greene-Kaufman, and Jae Shin all joined me in Seoul, which added dimensions and delight to my trip. Stefan Gehrman served as my research assistant and, among other tasks, compiled the data in the two appendices. Angela Miller, who has been my literary agent for many years, was, as always, generous with time, encouragement, apple butter, and books about Korea. Dr. Arthur Kleinman, Professor Michael Puett, and Jun Bum Sun provided insights into the philosophies that guide Korean life, in general, and K-drama, in particular. Douglas Farrand, Eugene Kim, and Dr. Margaux Simmons helped me understand the music of K-drama. Dr. Paul Browde helped me understand the "space between." Billy Kent explained the role of the soundtrack, which was a revelation.

I was supported by a sabbatical from The New School, which gave me time to study Korean, watch K-dramas, and travel to South

Korea. I am immensely grateful to President Kim Cassidy and Bryn Mawr College for the honor of the 2023 Flexner Lectureship. I presented three lectures on the Tao of K-drama, visited several classes, and participated in two conferences. I made new friends during that lovely process, including Professor Rhonda Hughes, Professor Isabel Lee, and Professor Tamarah Moss.

I am very grateful to the artists and designers who provided illustrations for this project. Mike Malbrough, our neighborhood friend whose art has inspired our work at the University of Orange for decades, did the drawings taken from screenshots and other photographs. These give the book its particular warmth. Audrey A. Jenkins's diagrams of infrastructures of care represent her exceptional analysis of that theme in CLOY. Aya Maruyama and Laura Van Vleet's map of Korea was made for our paper on the laundry in CLOY and helps us see the two countries of North and South Korea. William Morrish, my colleague at The New School, generously contributed two drawings that gave me a lot of focus. I am grateful to the *UE News* for permission to reprint the photo of my father at UE's 1954 Women's Conference. Rich Brown, who has helped me for many decades since he saved *Hillscapes: A Scrapbook* from ignominy, worked to get my drawings into presentable form.

I started this project in my living room, stuck and bored during the COVID shelter in place. It has been an experience beyond my wildest dreams, and I am deeply grateful to everyone, including all those not named here, who made it possible. All research is fraught with limitations and error, and cross-cultural research is especially vulnerable. All errors and misunderstandings are mine. I hope that they will all be corrected in time. And having finished this book, I am looking forward to writing in my 그림일기 (picture diary) again!

Identification and Confusion

"You feel me?"

—Javier Smith, author's grandson

"How could I be lonely when someone wrote a dictionary to understand me?"

—Jang So-young, *Mr. Queen*

Way-making (*dao*) is the flowing together of things (*wanwu*).

—*The Tao*, No. 62

I was a bit surprised to be asked to do a reading for my 1976 book, *Homeboy Came to Orange: A Story of People's Power*, as part of a 2025 book series in nearby Maplewood, New Jersey. It was a lively evening, and I shared lots of stories about the process of working with my father on his story. It is a wise book, and the struggles of 2025 had shown me that it had new lessons for us, as I explained to the audience. As we were leaving the venue, my granddaughter Lily Johnson pointed out that writing with my dad, who was struggling to finish his book in the last days of his life, was the foundation of my decades of work in narrative medicine.

This proposition startled me. My dad, Ernie Thompson, was then a 62-year-old former foundry worker who'd helped build his union, United Electrical Radio and Machine Workers of America (UE), during the Great Depression. His courage in facing the brutality of the capitalist factory owners was legendary, and he had a brusque, no-nonsense style acquired from those fights.

I was a 19-year-old college student, highly neurotic and self-absorbed, spending my time writing college papers by day and bad poetry by night. My dad and I had a highly conflictual relationship, as he thought I should be strong and I thought he should respect my feelings.

Our work on his book was quite an encounter. So much of his story went over my head. Simple statements like "I started to leaflet the factory next to my house" had no referent in my life, and I didn't understand that one until decades later, while driving in Hoboken with my mother, Maggie. She pointed to a brick condo we were passing and said, "That used to be a pencil factory that had been organized by UE and your dad was its business agent." There the former factory sat next to apartment buildings of the same vintage. I could (finally) see the mélange of the city my dad experienced. I grew up with an Olmsted park across the street rather than a factory next door.[1]

Because my job was to write what he described but what he described was incomprehensible to me, I got in terrible trouble over and over. "That's not what I said," he would yell at me; I would scream back at him and then cry to Mom that he was impossible.

But one day he told me a story about his work for women's rights and his role as the secretary of fair employment practices at UE. It was the summer of 1970, and women's liberation was everywhere. Dad and I had found common ground at last. This shared space expanded as he told me about his work with the National Negro Labor Council, which had led national struggles for equal opportunity in the workplace, desegregating Sears stores and the airlines, among others. With his permission, I decided to use that story for my senior honors thesis. He helped me connect with his colleagues near and far, including Coleman Young, who was then the mayor of Detroit (Figure I.1).[2]

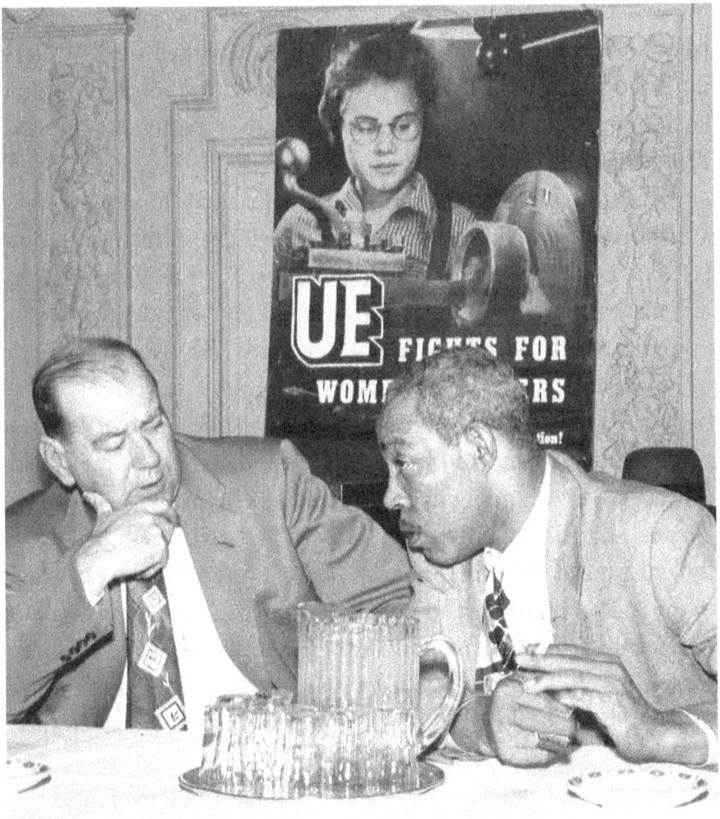

Figure I.1 Ernie at United Electrical, Radio, and Machine Workers of America (UE).
President Albert Fitzgerald confers with Ernest Thompson, secretary of the UE Fair Practices Committee, at the UE Women's Conference, 1954. Photograph from the *UE News*, used with permission.

Work on the book progressed steadily until one day it was done—and that same day, my dad died. I was crushed. Although I had revolted against his strictures for much of my childhood, we had become friends through working on the book. He may have been my best friend in that moment, and then he was gone. I couldn't face the final stages of work on the book. It stalled for five years, until Mom insisted I finish writing it. She took charge of editing, layout, and fundraising so it could be published by our imprint, Bridgebuilder Press, in 1976.[3]

I was in medical school at the time and focused on becoming a doctor. There are many kinds of doctoring, and medical school lays out a smorgasbord of enticing options. The first day of psychiatry clerkship a woman sat down and told me her story of growing up in the South in the last days of Jim Crow. Her vivid description of swimming in a creek and noticing a tapeworm coming out of her has stayed with me all these years. I became a psychiatrist because I thought I'd get to hear stories like that all the time. When I discovered I was going to be confined to a biomedical slice of the person—diagnosing illness and prescribing medicine (quickly)—I looked around for something else to do. It was 1986, the early days of the AIDS epidemic, and I got a new job studying excess risk for AIDS among Blacks and Hispanics in the United States. I found myself in a world of stories filled with addiction, death, trauma, and urban upheaval—so many stories and as many of them as I wanted to hear.

I have been listening to stories ever since and have found that my dad's insistence that I understand what he was saying, not what I thought he was saying, has rescued me over and over. As I grew as a listener, I learned to hear the multivocal chorus of voices that tell us stories of place. It is complex work, because a place is composed of the environment and the beings that live there: from nutty squirrels to old temples, they all have stories. It is thrilling work that has taken me to many places around the world.

That is, until COVID hit and my doctor sternly warned me to shelter in place. At home, alone, I found that I didn't want to read books; I wanted to watch television. But never having really paid attention to TV before, I lacked expertise. I had 300 channels on my cable TV. Though I had witnessed my grandchildren Lily and Javi move blithely among the channels, I had not mastered that skill. What I could do was press the "Netflix" button on my remote. There I found television from all over the world. And one day, Netflix suggested *Live Up to Your Name, Heo Im.*

This scene stands out in my mind: a Japanese soldier—after sneering at his homosexual general who had just released Heo Im and three other captives—casually lifts his rifle and fires at the fleeing group. A boy falls. The general curses. I knew in my bones what that scene was about.

In the next scene, Heo Im scoops up the child and pleads with a passing monk to take them in. With him are the boy's sister and Dr. Choi Yeon-kyung. Dr. Heo and Dr. Choi have been unsure about their feelings for each other, but they perform a surgery to remove the bullet in absolute synchrony. They are also able to see their own paths forward in a complicated world. The importance of this healing did not come into focus for me until a bit later in the show, when Heo Jun, Heo Im's mentor, told him that he had made progress toward enlightenment. "What?" I said. "When did that happen? How did that happen?"

It was a startling juxtaposition of identification and confusion, very much like my experiences with my father. The identification with *Live Up to Your Name* is rooted in the lived experience of our African American community. We have experienced wrenching oppression—being ripped from our homelands, forced into chattel slavery, denied our languages and customs, and, even after the end of slavery, engaged in the seemingly endless struggle between progress and regression. The look in the eyes of the Japanese soldier is one that is engraved in the souls of American Black people: police officers or racist attackers who looked at us in that way and casually—as if we had no humanity—pulled the trigger of their guns. That scene reads to me like my own history.

It is not just the sneer that resonates: the Japanese invasion signifies massive upheaval, which creates what I've called "root shock," the traumatic stress reaction to the loss of some or all of one's emotional ecosystem.[4] I knew, long before I read Korean history, that K-dramas were stories of root shock and upheaval.

But the confusion was equally profound. To the extent that "enlightenment" was a concept I'd encountered, it was something attained at the end of a serious commitment to meditation and mindfulness, none of which had been presented to us. I protested to the show, "What are you talking about?"

By that point in my life—January 2021—the space between getting it and not getting it was familiar territory to me, and I knew that exploring that space would offer huge rewards. I embarked on a course of study of K-drama, a genre of longform storytelling with shows that tell a complex story over 10 to 24 one-hour episodes. Between then and August 2025, I watched 88 K-dramas and studied Korean language, history, and culture. In 2023, I spent three months visiting South Korea.

My "reading" of K-drama came to pivot around the arc of the story, which is quite different from Western stories. K-dramas don't end with the lovers living happily ever after, with the redemption of the fallen person, or with the neurotic hero refusing to (pick one or more) grow up, sober up, try again, or take a chance on love—what we might call the not-happily-ever-after ending, which is, in many ways, the same thing.

K-drama follows what I call the arc of restoration, which moves from an opening catastrophe, through a period of recovery, onto engagement with the deeper wrong that triggered the events of the show. My beloved Dr. Heo Im, for example, was a miser who danced with his gold, because he resented that his consummate skill was not acknowledged with a prominent position close to the king. He was "a brat," as one of the characters in the show called him. Time travel and the love of a good woman straighten him out. Then Heo Im sees that the king is a coward after the king flees during the Japanese invasion of the Imjin War. It is the common people who step up to save the country. Heo Im joins their fight and begins to live up to his name—the name of the real man who was one of the most renowned acupuncturists of the Joseon era.[5]

Going Back

It was some time travel of my own that pulled together several threads in my life. In June 2021, Ruth Lindeborg, chief of staff at my alma mater, Bryn Mawr College, wrote to say,

> I write in hopes of scheduling a conversation with you about the Mary Flexner Lectureship, Bryn Mawr's most prestigious endowed lectureship and its oldest (established in 1928). The Flexner Lectureship has been held by many distinguished humanists and humanistic social scientists, beginning with Alfred North Whitehead in 1929; the most recent recipients have been Anthony Appiah (2005), Rashid Khalidi (2007), Sanjay Subrahamanyam (2009), Judith Butler (2011), Bonnie Honig (2017), and Fred Moten (2020–2021). President Cassidy hopes she might extend an invitation to you to be the next holder of the Flexner Lectureship, ideally sometime in the 2023–2024 academic year, and has asked me to explore that possibility with you.

This was truly a case of they "had me at hello." I wrote back something like "WOW!" and then said something along the lines of

> Oh, by the way, I am studying K-drama—my study is half a year old—and I would like to deliver the lectures on that. I have a sabbatical coming up and plan to go to Korea, so why not speak about this interest.

There was some hesitance of the "You're studying what?" variety, but eventually we agreed on this topic. I worked hard in the subsequent two years and hammered out the idea of the arc of restoration. I was excited about sharing it and didn't see what was coming. I should have. As I had written in my 2004 book *Root Shock*:

> Places are not simply bricks and mortar that provide us shelter. Because we dance in a ballroom, have a parade in a street, make love in a bedroom, and prepare a feast in a kitchen, each of these places becomes imbued with sounds, smells, noises, and feelings of those moments and how we lived them. When we enter an old classroom, the smell of chalk on the boards can bring back a swarm of memories of classmates and lessons, boredom and dreams.[6]

What Bryn Mawr gave me on those bright fall days in 2023, when I delivered the lectures, was a swarm of memories. Bryn Mawr's president Kim Cassidy pointed out that it's one thing to go to a reunion with your class—"It's like a theme park" was how she put it—and quite another to find a lawn chair and eavesdrop on the undergraduates' urgent discussions of getting drunk and hooking up.

Every bit of my highly neurotic college years came whooshing back to me. Of course, in those days, I read books and wrote papers, including one about the National Negro Labor Council, which continues to serve as a resource for scholars. But mostly I suffered and wondered how to find my way through. I remembered that I had discovered that I was *not* meant to be a doctor, that I was gifted at history and was excited for graduate school and a PhD. And I remembered that I didn't really have a senior year because much of the time I was at home, helping Dad finish *Homeboy*. When he died in January of that year, I sank into a grief so deep it took me a decade to emerge.

I dropped out of graduate school in 1971 and eventually wandered back into medicine, explaining to myself that it was the right career choice for me and I was just too young when I first tried the premed courses—all would be different the second time around.

My return to Bryn Mawr caused me to look back. Remembering my younger self groping for a path and choosing one that did and didn't make sense was devastating. My daughter Molly was emphatic that becoming a doctor was not a wrong choice. When President Cassidy asked at the midpoint of the lectureship if I were tired, I responded, "Yes, but I didn't expect the nervous breakdown."

My granddaughter (and mentor) Lily assured me that my nervous breakdown didn't show—that it was contained—but to me it seemed like the world was cracking up, throwing up memories and realities I'd never seen before. I mourned the career as a historian I never had, as well as all the challenges in medicine I did have.

The spiral of memory is a Great Power indeed. We do not live our lives in a straight line forward. Rather, we circle between what has been and what is to be. It is not a closed loop, but a spiral, meaning that remembering can be different, it can take us somewhere we have not yet been. Like the acupuncturist Heo Im, I found myself out of time and realized some very important things about that time of mourning and confusion. Among them was this big one: that the book I was helping my father write was a story of restoration. My dad, the homeboy, came to Orange, New Jersey, defeated by McCarthyism. His mourning was deep. My mother thought the cure for this would be to start organizing again, and she pointed out that the schools were segregated. That got him started. New friendships arose, which healed his wounds and gave him new hope. His organizing changed Orange for the better and helped generations of children in the city have a better future.

During my Flexner visits at Bryn Mawr I was able to see my father's story almost as a new narrative. Though knocked down by McCarthyism, he was able to rebuild his life, work with his new friends, and put a new pattern on our hometown. Lily's insight offered hope-filled clarity about the ways in which my life's work was grounded in my work with my dad—which did not end with his death on January 25, 1971, but has continued as the roots of my endeavors for all these decades.

K-Drama as Narrative Medicine

Narrative medicine puts forward the proposition that narratives are a fundamental tool for medicine, teaching us about illness and recovery by and with stories. K-dramas make a signal contribution to the world's literature on healing. I have several propositions to offer on this point.

The first is that K-dramas draw on the deep wisdom of the Korean people. Koreans have lived on the peninsula for thousands of years and during that time have developed a complex culture. They have withstood hundreds of invasions, fighting off would-be conquerors to preserve and maintain their way of life. They understand catastrophe and recovery because they have lived it and in that process have elaborated their insights.

The second proposition is drawn from the fact that K-dramas open with trauma. This trauma-informed storytelling has much to teach us about the nature of traumatic injury to the individual and the individual's community. A world awakening to the power of trauma to distort our lives is eager for knowledge about the sequelae of trauma in all its forms.

The third proposition is that K-drama's narrative arc is one of restoration. This narrative form is anchored in two concepts: that people can change and grow and that human beings put patterns on the world. We can change these patterns and therefore are not stuck in the "same old, same old." There are infinite possibilities inside the person, among the people, and in the societies in which we find ourselves. We can recover, we can work with others, and we can make a better place.

The fourth proposition is that K-drama enchants us because there is both emotional proximity and cultural distance, the contradiction I experienced with my dad all those years ago. In the case of K-drama, I believe that identification and confusion are essential to the worldwide popularity of this form, with its hundreds of millions of fans. On the one hand, I could identify with the pain caused by the Japanese invasion, while on the other hand, I couldn't see what they meant by progress toward enlightenment. This is simultaneously engaging, intriguing, and freeing: I'm hooked by the show and can't look away; at the same time, I can't take their word for it, as I have no idea what their word means. The identification and confusion create a space of exploration that I like a lot and I think many others do too. That is not to say that we all experience the same identification and the same confusion. A viewer in South Africa or Bolivia will have their own set of these two experiences, but I believe the combination holds enchantment for all of us.

The fifth proposition is that the method of storytelling is, in the words of my colleague Maura Spiegel, "intrinsically connected to its meaning." Professor Lily Ling, author of *The Dao of World Politics*, in discussing the many levels of narration in the Chinese classic *Dream of the Red Chamber*, noted that it "demonstrates Daoist dialectics not only in the story, but also in how it is told. [It] opens with four levels of narration, each signifying a 'world,' with protagonists transmuting back and forth . . . [a] constant telling and retelling, writing and rewriting, across these different worlds."[7] This "storytelling as movement" integrates "life as change" into the fabric of all we see. What will be revealed in the show is the manner in which traumatized people, through all the confusion, become able to see the Way, make the hard choices, and do the next right thing. The depiction of *becoming in the presence of noise* is the heart of the genre.

Following the Dialectic of He + She Becoming They

Mr. Queen illuminates this "becoming in the presence of noise." The show was extremely popular in Korea, and the rest of the world liked it too. The show's Wikipedia entry notes, "*Mr. Queen* took 5th place in the Netflix global viewing hours with 20.9 million viewing hours in its first week after it was made available for streaming on Netflix. It reached Top 10 in TV in 33 countries from Africa, Asia, and the Americas."[8]

In this K-drama, a tall, handsome, self-centered, womanizing master chef is framed for a crime and sought by the police. In seeking to escape, he falls into a pool, which becomes a lake. A woman swims toward him and kisses him. He emerges from the lake in the body of the beautiful queen to be, 200 years before his own time. He is shocked to have lost his genitals and frantic to get back to the future. His early efforts fail and he switches his tactics to ensure his own survival and avoid sex with the king, who is wooing him/her. His freewheeling style—an evolving combination of 21st-century uber-man and 19th-century aristocratic woman—shocks everyone around him. They want him to fit the mold of a woman of Joseon, and their repression acts like the bars of his cage, fueling the back-and-forth search for a way, which becomes the search for the Way.

Over time, the "he" of the beginning comes to think like the woman and feel the woman's attraction to the king. He even gives himself a hybrid name—combining her name, Kim So-young and his name Jang Bong-hwan into Kim Bong-hwan or Jang So-young. "He" who has, rather literally, become "they," rejects the Kim family, which made several attempts to murder him/her, and adopts the name Jang So-young. This is truly a show about transitioning, which resonates in the 2025 context of trans people as political scapegoats.[9]

Because Jang So-young is rocked back and forth between the limits of *his* self-concern and the possibilities of *their* being "all in" with the king, we see how social interaction supports the transition. As an example, they use many expressions from our times that their husband can't understand. The king deals with this by making a dictionary of the queen's language. As they grow closer and the transition has progressed, the king asks Jang So-young, "Are you lonely?" Jang So-young answers, "How could I be lonely when someone made a dictionary to understand me?" The king beams at them and they fall totally in love with their husband and go all in with him in the fight against those who would try to usurp the throne.

This is K-drama, so Jang Bong-hwan is wrenched back to the future, never (?) to see their beloved again. The shock of that is tempered by learning that what they taught their husband influenced the future of the nation and what they learned from him has rippled forward to change their 21st-century life for the better.

But do we know if *they* returned or just *he* came back? We don't.

What has become clear is what I call the "Tao of K-drama," the philosophical assumptions—the wisdom—that informed the story of a strange experience that pushed a selfish, self-seeking man to think of others more than himself, to follow a moral path, and to take comfort in love.

In the sense that K-dramas tell stories of healing, they hold seeds of healing for us, the viewers, in all the ways narratives work not only in medicine but also as medicine. Through our identification with the story, we can find solutions to our problems. Through our confusion, we can open up questions we need to answer. Through the experience of lovely storytelling, we can feel cheered and enchanted. In the case of K-drama, the arc of the narrative shifts from "happily ever after" to restoration, which has profound consequences for our ability to endure and grow.

The Organization of This Book

My goal in this book is to surface the several ways in which the wise narratives of K-drama achieve the intention of healing. I open each chapter with three quotes, the first representing my African American heritage, the second derived from a K-drama, and the third from *The Tao,* as translated by Roger Ames and David Hall.

Chapter 1, "*K-Drama Presents*: Stories of Restoration," discusses the core strategies K-drama uses to reveal the path from chaos to community.

Chapter 2, "The Town Shrink Watches Carefully," outlines the recovery tasks that underlie the arc of restoration.

Chapters 3 to 9 examine K-dramas, each selected to represent a particular level of social organization, because healing must occur at each of these levels to make society and its members whole. Old Master Lao Tzu, who is credited as the author of *The Tao,* described the systems and their nested relationship in this manner:

> If there is to be peace in the world,
> There must be peace in the nations.
> If there is to be peace in the nations,
> There must be peace in the cities.
> If there is to be peace in the cities,
> There must be peace between neighbors.
> If there is to be peace between neighbors,
> There must be peace in the home.
> If there is to be peace in the home,
> There must be peace in the heart.

In the US, people tend to simplify this construction to the final line—peace in the heart—which leads to the conclusion, "I should meditate." But K-drama has a much deeper understanding of the Old Master's implicit "and" between each of the levels. Each of these seven chapters focuses on a particular K-drama, chosen because its plot is located at a particular level of scale of the social world and, following Old Master Lao Tzu's intention, lets us see the other levels as we move among the storylines.

Chapter 3, "Peace in the Heart: Heo Im Gets Sent to the School of Hard Knocks," is focused on a suffering individual's achievement of "peace in the heart." It explores the story of Heo Im, a beleaguered and bratty acupuncturist who has strayed from the path and must be set right. As per the story's title, Heo Im is admonished to *Live Up to Your Name*! In my African American tradition people say, "The School of Hard Knocks is a tough school, but a fool will learn in no other." That is where Heo Im gets sent so he can get his head on straight.

Chapter 4, "Peace in the Home: Cha Eun-ho Gets a Roommate," focuses on *Romance Is a Bonus Book*, the story of Kang Dan-i, who finds herself homeless, shoeless, penniless, unemployed, and caught in the rain without an umbrella. Cha Eun-ho, her best friend, asks her, "Where are you?" and she replies, "I'm at the edge of my life." Peering through the curtains at Dan-i's burgeoning romance with that dear friend, we watch as they make a peaceful home and better workplace.

Chapter 5, "Peace in the Neighborhood: Kim Je-hyeok Builds a Team," is situated among neighbors inside and outside a prison. It looks at the troubles of Kim Je-hyeok, a famed baseball player who is imprisoned for assault. In the US this show is called *Prison Playbook*, while in Korean it is known as *Wise Prison Life*. It examines the ways in which the love of the people around him helps Kim Je-hyeok both learn the lesson he is supposed to learn and become able to help others as well.

Chapter 6, "Peace in the City: Lee Gang-du Re-members a City," takes us to the city level and shows peacemaking at that scale. It looks at the way in which Lee Gang-du, who survived a building collapse in his early teens, is able to move out of his own trauma to ensure that the replacement building will be built to code and honor the memories of those lost in the tragedy. The US name of the show, *Rain or Shine,* gives nothing away, but the Korean title, *Just Between Lovers*, gets to the heart of the matter.

Chapter 7, "Peace in the Nation: Dam-i Takes on Evil," takes us to the level of the nation, in the show *The King's Affection.* We meet Dam-i, a princess with a strong moral code who is forced to masquerade as her murdered brother. Though living a lie, she fights for justice and takes on her evil grandfather in a fight to the death.

Chapter 8, "Peace in the World: Captain Ri Crosses the Line," explores the partition of Korea by taking South Korean heiress Yoon Se-ri into the demilitarized zone, where she falls into the arms of Captain Ri of the North Korean army, literally *Crash Landing on You*, as the title says. Their love will force them to confront the most rigid boundary in the world and will teach us about the international system that maintains it. When Captain Ri steps over that boundary, he shows us that we can take small chances for the sake of peace.

Chapter 9, "Peace Between the Universes: Lee Gon Is in Time," examines a show called *The King: Eternal Monarch.* This K-drama moves into the interdimensional space to explore two Koreas, one that is the Kingdom of Corea, which experienced neither Japanese colonialism nor the Korean War, and one that is the Republic of Korea we know today. Like all the leading figures, King Lee Gon is tormented by his past but must use those experiences to save the worlds threatened by his traitorous uncle.

Chapter 10, "Tides of Hope," explores the effect of having a new view of my own life as well as the ways in which this helped me be a better teacher.

We all dwell in confusion at this moment in history. That is where the wisdom of K-drama comes to our aid: we all need this wisdom in these precarious times. K-drama feels precious to me because it brings a new solution. It is not my would-be heroic lone self that has to save the world. Rather, it is the community of all of us that will do that work. And we can start to build that power by reconnecting with one friend and walking together, accompanied by our stories and the stories that inspire us, on a path of collective recovery.

1

K-Drama Presents

Stories of Restoration

> To restore what has been torn apart, we must reweave the social fabric and reknit the physical spaces. We tell stories of restoration so that we know these efforts work.
>
> —Molly Kaufman, author's daughter

> "Your Highness, where have you been?"
> "In a place with a warm heart, Samdal-ri."
>
> —Courtier and his prince, *Welcome to Samdal-ri*

> It is simply in doing things noncoercively (*wuwei*)
> That everything is governed properly.
>
> —*The Tao*, No. 3

Restoration stories resonate during these troubled times precisely because they are not about individual triumph over disaster but rather about groups rising to meet a challenge. In times when worldwide upheaval is causing deepening despair and disorientation, these stories give us hope, help us look in new directions, and teach about an etiquette of belonging that most of us in the Western world never learned.

Although individualism has been a source of creativity and invention for centuries, we are in desperate need of restoration stories because unbridled "me me me" thinking has gotten us into a boatload of trouble, like our rapidly changing climate and the spread of authoritarianism. As Albert Einstein pointed out, we can't solve a problem with the thinking that created it—we have to change our thinking, particularly how we think on our feet and act. To do that, many things will have to happen, some of which are hard and others of which are not so hard.

Research in mental health has shown that massive changes in emotions and behaviors will follow cognitive shifts of the "glass half empty/glass half full" sort. Both statements are true of a glass filled to the middle, but the consequences of choosing one over the other are not the same. If I can choose the positive statement, I will feel better. And frankly, it's not that hard to teach or learn. I am proposing that groups too can use a cognitive approach to shift behavior. Specifically, if we can see and name the arc of restoration, we have a vision of the future toward which we can work.

In the final year of his life, the Reverend Dr. Martin Luther King Jr. posed the question "Where do we go from here?" Dr. King thought it was evident that we were creating chaos but that we had the opportunity to take a new path. Sadly, we continued on the path toward chaos, and now we find ourselves at a very difficult point. But if we understand that change is the only constant, then we also know that the current state of things is not fixed. We can get back to the main road, the Way of Tao. We can put new patterns on the world that will work better for us. We can go from chaos to community and thereby save ourselves and all the species that evolved with us. With that in mind, I propose that K-drama's narrative propositions—its arc of restoration, pattern language, and ways of showing community—offer us that cognitive shift and new possibilities for healing.

The Arc of Restoration

The storyline in K-drama addresses two levels of repair: (1) the traumatized protagonist and (2) the social organization that

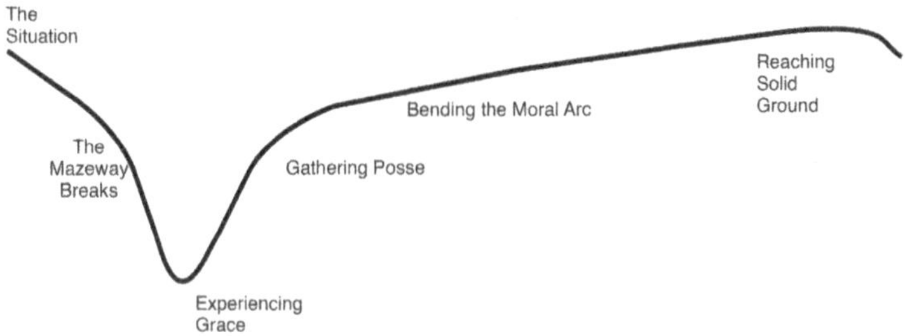

Figure 1.1 Arc of Restoration.
This diagram demonstrates the narrative path of K-drama from the opening situation to the closing attainment of solid ground.

produced the trauma. I have identified six phases of the arc of restoration (Figure 1.1).

The shows always open with a "situation," in the most dire sense of "We have a situation here." Agatha Christie titled one of her novels *A Murder Is Announced*, which is in the spirit of K-drama openers. Hence, the opening part of the arc of restoration is "the situation."

Because of the situation, the logic of the known world, the mazeway, has broken and the protagonists are left carrying a heavy, and perhaps paralyzing, burden of confusion and trauma. A moment of grace will open space for breathing and reconnecting. Then the protagonists are able to pull together a group of friends—a posse—that can tackle the social issues, bend the moral arc toward justice, and reach solid ground. We have not returned to the place from which we started. Instead, we have put a new pattern on the world.

In *Welcome to Samdal-ri*, we can see a particularly precious unfolding of this arc. The present is shaped by an old tragedy, the drowning of a *haenyo*, one of the female divers who harvest seafood off the coast of Jeju Island in Korea. Her husband can't forgive her best friend and fellow haenyo for her death. The women's children, Cho Sam-dal and Cho Yong-pil, were born on the same day and have been twinned since birth. However, their love for each other has been derailed by Cho Yong-pil's father's unresolved resentment.

Into this complex setting comes "the situation." As a young girl, Cho Sam-dal tells a variety show host that she heard that dragons rise from small streams, and she wants to be a dragon. He says, "Oh, you want to go to Seoul?" Cho Sam-dal makes it to Seoul and succeeds, but a jealous employee sets out to destroy her. Cho Sam-dal has to retreat to Jeju to escape hordes of reporters eager to defame her. The central metaphor in the show is that the free-diving haenyos are taught not to be greedy and to return to the surface when they can't hold their breath anymore. The headline of the trailer is "The Big Fish Returns to Catch Her Breath."

Back in Jeju, the simmering past and boiling present collide, leaving Cho Sam-dal frantic. How will things slow down so she can breathe? I would place the moment of grace in her first face-to-face encounter with her estranged beloved, Cho Yong-pil. He mistakes her for an intruder and calls friends over to help him subdue the interloper. Just as the friends are arriving, Cho Yong-pil realizes that it is Cho Sam-dal. He can see that she is terrified the friends will see her, so he takes a piece of cloth and fans it out to cover her. The rise of the lightweight, translucent cloth, with sun shining through, and its gentle descent to drape her body create a moment apart, a moment of being protected instead of attacked. Terror is replaced by safety. It is a short moment, but that is the nature of such moments of grace in K-drama. It is enough to permit the restoration to begin.

While Cho Sam-dal and Cho Yong-pil have much to overcome, they will not do it alone. They will need friends, family, and the surrounding village to break open Cho Yong-pil's father's frozen rage, keep the howling press off Cho Sam-dal, and get the young people on their way. The resolution of the multiple problems is not accomplished through grand gestures but rather through a "microprocess" of small interactions. For example, the deceased haenyo's mother, now an old woman with dementia, has a moment of clarity. She puts her hand on that of her embittered son-in-law and says, "Don't have resentment."

He slowly gets what she's saying and is stunned.

As he opens his mind a little, he is able to ask Cho Sam-dal's mother and his wife's best friend whom he's blamed all these years, "When do you miss her most?"

She promptly answers, "When I dive into the sea or see her son."

He walks away without a word, but his worldview has again been challenged. These small moments accumulate until his prison of grief and jealousy breaks open. Then he and Cho Sam-dal's mother are freed.

The title of the 15th episode is "It Takes a Village to Raise a Dragon." This has the double meaning of helping the young dragon grow up and lifting the dragon into the air so it can fly to its destiny. The "village"—the collective—supplies the power for the lift. Cho Sam-dal is being hunted by reporters. The villagers refuse to tell the reporters where she lives, sending them on a vain quest for their prey. While the reporters are out of the way, the villagers help Cho Sam-dal reclaim her career by putting on an exhibition of her photos of the people of the village. The parallel processes of healing the old resentment and restoring the young dragon to the sky bend the moral arc of the universe toward justice. Cho Sam-dal, Cho Yong-pil, and their friends are freed to go to Seoul where they find new success in their chosen careers.

A foreigner, Kim Man-su, who was working in the village convenience store, sums up the show for us. He suddenly leaves Samdal-ri, giving the village a billion-won gift. We later see him walking in the garb of an Arab prince and one of his entourage asks, "Your Highness, where have you been?"

"In a place with a warm heart," he replies, "Samdal-ri."

The Pattern Language

K-drama speaks through a pattern language of human relationships, what many observers refer to as "tropes." The architect Christopher Alexander studied organic forms of architecture around the world and discovered that there were common solutions to many challenges of organizing space.[1] The solution for creating an attractive entrance, for example, was echoed across cultures. These he called "patterns," and he noted that there were patterns at every level of scale—the house, the block, the neighborhood, the city, and the nation. These taken together created a "language" of spatial organization that was aesthetically accessible and functional for people's daily lives.

Telling stories of complex situations produces a "pattern language" as well. While to my knowledge no one has produced a dictionary of situations in the sense and spirit of Alexander's book, we have encoded them in words, of which we have thousands. To list just a few of my favorites: kidnapped, ambushed, marooned, divorced, remarried, outgunned, imperiled, and immigrated. Architect William Morrish, who studied with Alexander while at UC Berkeley, particularly loves "ambush." "Life is always an ambush!" he declares.

I learned about pattern language in K-drama by seeing one in a show and then encountering it again in the Passover Seder.

> In the K-drama *Misaeng: Incomplete Life*, a show about office life, the young and vulnerable Jang Geu-rae is ambushed by Mr. Park, his sleazy superior. Mr. Park harasses Jang Geu-rae with withering comments and unseemly demands. Jang Geu-rae is obviously hurt but does not resist. As the camera pans around the nearby cubicles, we see the pained faces of the other people in the office who can hear and see what's going on.[2]
>
> Jang Geu-rae's horrified superior, Kim Dong-shik, takes him aside and asks him why he's just going along with the abuse: he clearly has the right to fight back. In response, Jang Geu-rae confides that he trained as a professional Go player and is using a Go strategy that entails fighting back by holding his position, thus creating a countercurrent against his opponent.

When I saw the distress on the faces of Jang Geu-rae's coworkers as they witnessed Park's effort to degrade Jang Geu-rae, his nonaggressive strategy made sense to me. By the time Jang Geu-rae exposes Mr. Park as a criminal, everyone understands what is going on. They do not try to protect Mr. Park. Rather, they are relieved to see his evil ways exposed. The loss of connection and social support was the end of Mr. Park, who was fired and arrested for his criminal activity.

This is a very satisfying story, which I presented at a talk I gave in South Korea. A few days later, I used Zoom to join the Passover Seder with my Unitarian Universalist congregation in Orange, New Jersey. The service includes reading about Moses's demands of Pharaoh to "let my people go." Part of the biblical story is confusing. On the one hand, God tells Moses to make this demand of Pharaoh, while on the other hand God "hardens Pharaoh's heart" so that Pharaoh says "no" the first nine times Moses comes before him. I'm not the only one puzzled by this: theologians have pondered this for millennia.

This time, while listening to that part of the Seder, I had the niggling thought, "Wait, I've just heard this story somewhere else." Later that day, I realized that it was Jang Geu-rae who'd shown me this strategy. In that case, Jang Geu-rae held his position, accepting the horrible orders of his superior and creating the conditions to bring Mr. Park to justice. And K-drama shows us what the conditions are; as the camera pans across the cubicles and we see the coworkers' distress and disgust, we know that no one is going to defend Mr. Park—they can't wait to see him go.

While trying to free the Jews, Moses holds his position. He asks for liberation, while Pharoah—under God's compulsion—says no, no, no, no. Having seen *Misaeng*, I can fill in the part of the story that the Bible left out. What we realize is that other people—besides Moses and Pharoah—are living through this situation too.

Knowing how people are, we can imagine that most people shrugged off the water turning to blood.

Then Pharaoh said no again and there were frogs. So, OK, frogs.

Then Pharaoh said no again—lice—well, that got a little more personal. And a plague of flies—get out of my face! God is upping the ante, which cuts through people's tolerance and their defenses—they're getting annoyed and they're talking to one another. "Can you believe what's happening?"

"No, I can't."

"Can't he just let them go?"

"Well, letting go of the slaves—who'll do the work? You?"

But then Pharaoh says no again and the livestock start to die.

People are getting frightened—the escalation continues. Finally, when we reach the death of the newborn, no one can take it anymore, not even Pharoah. All the Egyptians and all the Jews are on the same page—Let the Jews go!

And so Pharaoh said yes and the Jews were free.

This made me wonder about the knowledge of the countercurrent strategy back in those times. It turns out that Go was invented about 4,000 years ago in China,[3] and the Exodus occurred approximately 1446 BCE, or 3,466 years ago.[4] Thus, the knowledge of the countercurrent strategy had been worked out in the ancient world and was likely known to both Go players and those writing the Torah (and God, of course). My granddaughter Lily pointed out that the countercurrent strategy wouldn't work if we were not, in reality, all connected.

This is an example of a particularly complex and arcane pattern, but once I had seen it in K-drama and recognized it at Seder, I began to notice the many variations that abound in daily life. Waiters, for example, practice this strategy, accepting the rudeness of one table while winning admiration and big tips from tables nearby. I'm sure more examples will come to mind as you look for this in your daily life. It would not be good to respond to every ambush in this way, but it is helpful to know you might be able to use the countercurrent strategy in the right circumstance.

The Language of Community

Watching the improbable stories of K-drama, we see versions of very real, very human situations. By showing people work through them, K-drama enriches our vocabulary in the pattern language of restoration. This cognitive shift from isolated hero to struggle in community is fundamental to our restoration—it gives a new mindset with which to find solutions to our problems.

K-dramas are telling these stories of restoration by working in the web of connection, which is multidimensional and encompasses all time and space. K-dramas shift to the past in order to reveal the backstory of the characters, and then they return to the present to examine the unfolding of the current situation. They alternate among cities and among spaces in cities. They may use time travel to move characters back and forth across epochs. And there are always multiple storylines. Through the multiplicity and mixing of storylines, we are brought into the complexity of the world.

Learning to follow so many storylines was difficult for me and reminded me of a seminal experience early in my research on urban renewal. In 1995 I read a special section of the *Roanoke Times and World News* written by Mary Bishop, which told the story of the destruction of several Black neighborhoods in that city.[5] She quoted many people, and I asked myself why it was necessary to tell the story through so many voices? Soon after I read the article, I went to visit Mary in Roanoke, Virginia. She showed me all around the neighborhoods that had been affected, as well as the larger city. She introduced me to people who had lived through the terrible destruction of their homes and neighborhoods. Each place had a unique story, as did each person. I came to understand that no one voice could have told the story: it required a chorus.

And that is the premise of K-drama: to tell the stories of community, you need many sets of people and freedom to move in time and space.

In Season 2 of *Dr. Romantic*, one of the young doctors, Seo Woo-jin, pushes teacher Kim Sabu. He knows something is wrong with Dr. Kim. Dr. Kim loves this young man and accepts his rather desperate need to know. But, of course, he is Kim Sabu, so he shoves armsful of notebooks filled with journal articles at Seo Woo-jin. "You can ask one question," Dr. Kim barks.

Seo Woo-jin wonders what he's going to do—all the notebooks are named "The Cornered Stone Project." Does he have to read every article in every book? Fortunately, by this time in his work in Doldam Hospital, he has connected with three others, and together they start to work on the problem. One points out that the notebooks have different annotations, "GS" for General Surgery, "CS" for Cardiovascular Surgery, etc. "Dr. Kim said it didn't involve surgery, so we can eliminate those," the colleague suggests. This boils it down to one notebook—Neurology—it is almost immediately obvious what Dr. Kim's diagnosis is; I'm so indoctrinated in HIPAA that I feel like I can't say it here. But Seo Woo-jin goes back to Dr. Kim and names it. He is, indeed, correct.

We also learn what "The Cornered Stone Project" is—it is the effort of Dr. Kim and the hospital team to reflect on every case, learning from experience what succeeded and what might be done better. Throughout the series Dr. Kim has "known" things that others didn't—he says it's not intuition; it's unceasing study. Young Dr. Seo is invited to join the project, helping the hospital perfect its ability to serve.

Go, called "Baduk" in Korea, is played in a number of K-dramas, so I know that a "cornered stone" is one that is surrounded by the opposition. In *Captivating the King*, the fate of a cornered stone is a point of contention between the king and his *gidaeryeong*, Kang Mong-woo, the king's personal Baduk opponent (and beloved, need I say?). While the king is willing to sacrifice the cornered stone, Kang Mong-woo says that the cornered stone can always be saved, if you pay attention, and that this is the surer road to victory.

The metaphor of the cornered stone brings up that tension between abandoning the stone or finding a solution. *Dr. Romantic*'s Kim Sabu called on his community to save "the stone," meaning all the people seeking care in their emergency department. Then the community could rally around Seo Woo-jin to understand their leader's illness. In that process, they learn that he is now a cornered stone and they face the choice of abandonment or salvation. It wouldn't be K-drama if they didn't rally around him, showing us how to respond to threat as a well-integrated community.

Thus, the form—a situation played out over 16 episodes, with multiple storylines that take us backward and forward in the space and time of the web of connection as good and evil wrestle with each other—shows us how the arc of restoration moves us from chaos to community. And I knew, from my work and the work of my students, that people changed.

Audrey Jenkins was a student in my 2021 "Situation Analysis Through the Lens of K-Drama" class, which analyzed *Crash Landing on You*.[6] She became fascinated by the concept of care. The class had made a detailed analysis of each character in each episode, using the database software Airtable. Jenkins created a set of variables of care, which ranged from "genuine care" to "anti-care." She used Airtable to capture the kinds of caring actions each character took. As you can see in Figure 1.2, there is a great deal of change in what people feel and do. In the first episode, there is an equal division among the three variables, care for others ("we" care), self-care ("I" care), and anti-care. By the final episode, this

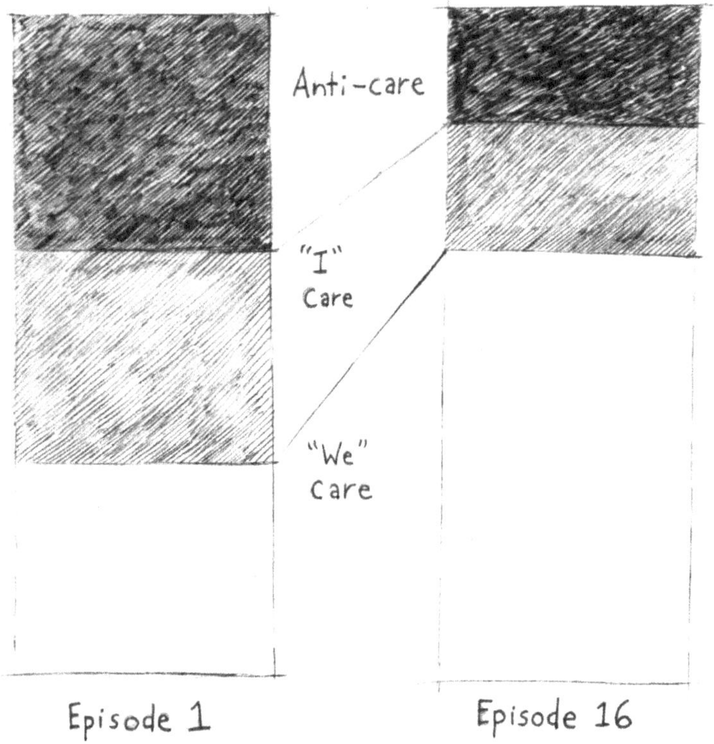

Figure 1.2 "We" Care.
This diagram shows the shift in the kinds of caring actions that are observed in the first and last episodes of *Crash Landing on You*. "Anti-care" actions are harmful, "I care" actions are concerned solely with the self, while "We care" actions help the group prosper.

has shifted, so that two-thirds of the characters are acting from "we" care.

Jenkins's precise analysis helps us see that people shift but begs the question, *what exactly happens to create change*? It took a new kind of analysis for me to answer that question.

2

The Town Shrink Watches Carefully

> Wherever you are, love is always there in the sky watching you.
>
> —Lily Johnson, author's granddaughter

> Buddhism, Taoism, Confucianism and Christianity are the superstructure of Korean thought, but the substructure is Shamanism.
>
> —Jun Bum Sun, author and ecologist

> Refined notes and raw sounds harmonize with each other,
> And before and after lend sequence to each other—
> This is really how it all works.
>
> —*The Tao*, No. 2

My friend Robert Sullivan took me to lunch one day and asked if he might write an article about me for *The New York Times Magazine.* When it came out in 2015, the headline was this: "The Town Shrink: Trained as a Psychiatrist, Mindy Thompson Fullilove Now Puts Entire Cities on the Couch."[1]

"Ha-ha," you might say, "K-drama put Mindy Fullilove on the couch."

And it put me to work on new questions, I would add. Early on in residency, I became convinced that change was hard for people—we get locked into our way of life, and even when this way of life is clearly harmful to us, we have a hard time shifting to a new way of life. Family therapy fascinated me because a shift in a family changes the behavior of many people. A major part of my training in family therapy was to watch videos of therapy as a teacher helped us "see" the kink in the family process so that we might envision the steps to change and ways to help people take them.

Looking at K-drama, I could see that people changed, but unlike my experience in family therapy training, the writers weren't stopping the show to decipher the process for me. I had to do that for myself. I had to watch very carefully. Interpersonal processes are subtle, and cultures differ in the ways in which people embody emotions. I was lucky to have my Korean language teacher Professor Kyla Park by my side, especially when I knew the subtleties of the language had not made it into the subtitles I was reading. Fellow psychiatrist Arthur Kleinman and his colleague Professor Michael Puett, as well as Korean friends Professor Eunju Hwang, artist and gardener Byun Jeong Dae-seob, and musician and writer Jun Bum Sun, also played major roles in steering this part of my inquiry.

A Worldview of Constant Change

K-drama arises from a worldview that is unlike ours, one that incorporates incessant change into everyday thinking and puts restoration into the context of thousands of years of history.

Dr. Kleinman, who has done a major portion of his work in China, oriented me to Asian philosophies, knowledge systems, and social practices. He urged me to read *The Path*, a book about ancient Chinese philosophers, and to speak with his colleague, its first author, Dr. Michael Puett, a professor of anthropology and Chinese history. Coauthored with Christine Gross-Loh, the book describes the work of Old Master Lao Tzu (6th century BCE), Confucius (551–479 BCE), Mozi (470–391 BCE), Mencius (4th century BCE), Xunzi (3rd century BCE), and others.[2] It is from that book that I learned about the philosophers of the Warring States period (475–221 BCE) in China, a time as trying as our own when philosophers searched for ways to live a good life in the face of chaos. They studied the dialectic—the yin-yang of the universe—and taught that nothing ever stands still or completely alone. Indeed, the connections among things are such that one becomes another in a constant, oscillating process of evolution and transformation. Mencius, for example, thought that accepting the instability of the world was foundational to clear thinking:

> Hard work would not necessarily lead to prosperity. Bad deeds would not necessarily be punished. There were no guarantees of anything; no stable, overarching coherence to the world that one could count on. Instead, Mencius believed, the world is fragmented, in perpetual disorder, and in need of constant work. And it is only when we understand that nothing is stable that we can make decisions and live our lives in the most expansive way.[3]

Given that worldview of constant change, there are three key lessons I took from my readings. The first lesson was to do nothing coercive. This is from Old Master Lao Tzu's *The Tao*, translated as "The Way." In our times "Tao" is a widely used synonym for wisdom. *The Tao* urges us to stay on the path. In many English translations, this is accompanied by the advice to "do nothing." "Staying on the path" is an action, and "doing nothing" was not an action—two pieces of advice I found contradictory. I was relieved to read in Roger Ames and David Hall's philosophical translation that "do nothing" is an "unfortunate" choice for translating *wuwei*. Rather, they say, *The Tao* urges us to do nothing *coercive*.[4]

This makes perfect sense in the active world of K-drama, in which the good people are not coercive and the evil people coerce others all the time. At least for the purposes of my study of K-drama, I believe that "do nothing coercive" is an instruction for staying in the Way.

Second, staying on the Path requires the cultivation of people. Mencius and others saw people as "under construction" throughout their lives, beings with a natural endowment of goodness that would emerge with cultivation. Enacting goodness, even in small behaviors and interactions with others, was essential both to being a person of character in an uncertain world and to making a world that was most supportive for all. One of Mencius's ideas seems to me to have particular salience in this regard. He observed that we feel a tingle of delight when we do something good for another person, including small acts like holding the door. These were "sprouts of goodness" that could grow. Puett and Gross-Loh note,

> You begin as a lone farmer, cultivating your sprouts in your humble field, but the effect radiates outward. Those on the receiving end of our goodness become inspired to act better and to continue growing their own sprouts of goodness in turn. Such moments of goodness build until they fill a day, and eventually an entire life.[5]

Confucius developed this thesis with a focus on the heart-mind. I had always thought of Confucianism as a rigid system that was the justification of hierarchy during feudalism. Artist Lee Kyungho, whom I met while visiting Tongdosa, a Buddhist monastery, assured me that the ideas of K-drama were more the legacy of Confucianism than Buddhism. This challenged my ideas about the two, and I asked Professor Puett to comment on this. He answered that state-sponsored Confucianism was what I was associating with Confucianism. But, he said, there was another aspect of Confucianism, which had to do with showing care, building and rebuilding community, and resisting coercion from greed and other evils. It was those aspects of Confucianism that resonated strongly with my own observations of K-drama.

Professor Puett also explained the importance of "heart-mind," the concept that the seat of emotions and the center of rationality are one. It is the use of our cognitive abilities to understand our emotions that allows us to cultivate the heart-mind, and in turn, it is the heart-mind that supports sound decision-making. In *The Path*, I found this important quote:

> Cultivating the heart-mind is an outwardly directed act intended not to remove us from the world but to engage more deeply in it so that we can better ourselves and everyone around us through every interaction. It is about paying attention not in a mindful way but a Confucian one.[6]

Third, I encountered the possibility of building and rebuilding in the work of Xunzi, who lived at the end of the Warring States period. Xunzi argued that people put patterns on the world, and we have the capacity to look at the pattern and evaluate it. If it is not working to make life better for us, we have the ability to change it. Xunzi proposed:

> Heaven and Earth gave birth to us. We give pattern to Heaven and Earth. We form a triad with Heaven and Earth, are the summation of the myriad things, and the father and mother of the people. Without us, Heaven and Earth have no pattern.[7]

Puett and Gross-Loh comment, "If we have made the world that we experience, then we should not be asking ourselves how to find our proper place within it. We should be asking whether we structured it well."[8]

Thus, we arrive at four proposals for action in a world that is capricious and ever-changing:

- Do nothing coercive.
- Do acts of goodness.
- Cultivate heart-mind.
- Put patterns on the world that serve us.

Watching the Contradictions

My father Ernie taught me that change was the only constant, though, of course, as a know-it-all teenager, I didn't believe him. He also taught me that to read change, I needed to study the contradictions. "Taught" is a little extreme, as his method of "teaching" was to say, "Read the book" while walking out of the room. The "book" was Chairman Mao's pamphlet *On Contradiction.* Mao was not fabulously more patient than my father, and I got stuck almost immediately. Mao wrote, "The absoluteness of contradiction has a twofold meaning. One is that contradiction exists in the process of development of all things, and the other is that in the process of development of each thing a movement of opposites exists from beginning to end."[9]

Obviously, Chairman Mao thought of those two statements as different, but as a 16-year-old, I could not fathom how that might be. I read those lines over and over for a couple of years before the idea yielded itself to me. The first concept asserts that there are contradictions in the development of all things. In the development of a living being, for example, there is a contradiction between life and death. In the rise of an autocrat, in another example, there is a contradiction between the autocrat's ability to impose his will and the people's desire to be free.

The second concept is that the tension between the contradictions is not static. A living being is full of vigor at the beginning of life, but that life force weakens over time. Eventually the being will die. Similarly, autocrats, if they hold enough power, can start out getting their own way. But the power of the people will be a force resisting the autocrat, and that force will grow over time. Eventually, the autocrat will be overthrown.

Once I understood these two fundamental concepts, I found that it was helpful to look for contradictions in the world around me. At the time, I was organizing against the war in Vietnam. The tension between the "good life" in the US and the "destruction" of Vietnam was always there. Initially, not too many people knew what was happening in Vietnam because of the war, and it was easier to dismiss concerns about it. As the costs of the war started to undermine the "good life" in the US, more people paid attention and were shocked by what we were doing. This ultimately turned people against the war, and the US government was forced to withdraw.

When I started to study acupuncture during residency, I learned about yin and yang, states of energy we might say, and these lend a new character to the aspects of the contradiction. The autocrat, when seizing power, is full of yang, and the people who are under his heel are quite yin. But these states will change over time. Adding heart-mind to this, we can rewrite the arc of restoration to show that the early, downward phase of a show is the period of the yin of good and the yang of evil. After the heart-mind is opened by grace, we enter the second, upward phase of the yang of good and the yin of evil. Bill Morrish, adding a baseline to my original arc of restoration and writing heart-mind as "HeartMind," drew it for me (Figure 2.1).

SmallGestures, Big Change

So, how *do* people change?

What the philosophers—Lao Tzu, Confucius, Mencius, Xunzi, Thompson, and Mao—taught had to be connected to what I was

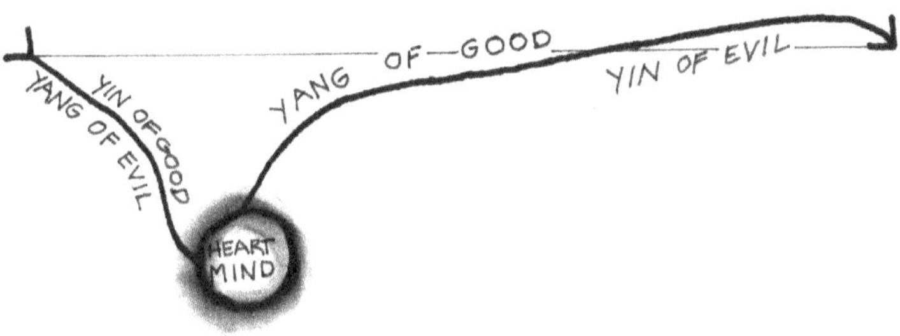

Figure 2.1 Yin-Yang in the Narrative Arc of K-Drama.
The movement of opposites follows a pattern in the narrative arc of K-drama, with evil in its yang phase at the beginning but yin at the end, and the opposite for good. The pivot happens at the HeartMind.
Drawing by William Morrish, used with permission.

actually seeing on television. On the one hand, we have the forces of evil. Per *The Tao*, they are the people who carry sharp swords and have more than they need. These forces are constantly trying to take from the people. They have characteristic "tells," as poker players might call them: the snarl of a lip, the hand raised to hit, the spiteful voice, the cold eyes that accompany a lifeless smile. Because every show has a villain, we get a lot of opportunities to see how they act, and it is shown with the same attention to detail as is applied to showing trauma and recovery.

On the other hand, we have the forces of good, the people who hope to create a pattern of sharing and mutual aid. The work of good is embodied in these SmallGestures that people make: (1) "pull your coat"; (2) show micro-kindnesses; (3) stand in the face of love; (4) do the next right thing, which bends the moral arc of the universe; and (5) have a party.

SmallGestures: "Pull Your Coat"

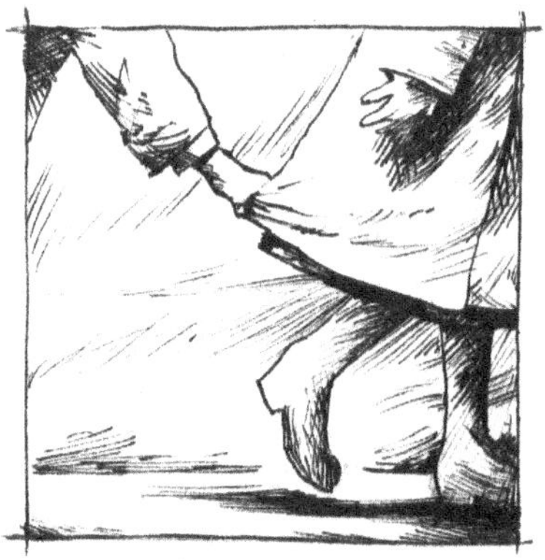

Figure 2.2 SmallGesture: Pull Your Coat.
A hand tugs at a coat.
Drawing by Mike Malbrough, used with permission.

One of my father Ernie's favorite expressions was "pull your coat," as in "He pulled your coat" (Figure 2.2). A lot of African American speech is metaphorical, and this is on purpose: it is not easily decipherable—one has to be initiated into it, and one has to be old enough to understand metaphor, past the concrete interpretations of imagining someone pulling my coat. The time came when I could get the figurative meaning, that pulling your coat meant to pull you back from risk, from stupidity, from danger.

In the K-drama *Once Upon a Small Town*, Han Ji-yool, a young veterinarian, goes to the countryside to mind his grandfather's practice. He meets Ahn Ja-young, the delightful village police officer, but can't readily admit to himself that he likes her. So he is rude to her—that he can so easily express his anger toward her reflects shades of patriarchy, an underlying and unresolved issue of the story—but his nine-year-old neighbor, Lee Sang-hyeon, chastises him and hands him his phone so he can apologize: the boy pulls his coat and gets him on the right path.

SmallGestures: Kindness

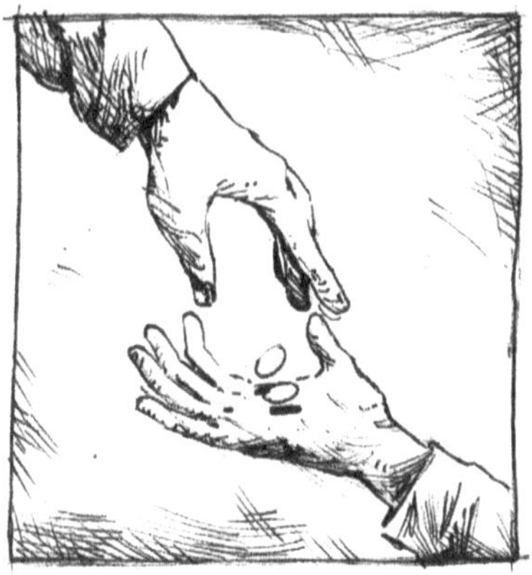

Figure 2.3 SmallGesture: Kindness. A hand held out for help is receiving coins from another hand.
Drawing by Mike Malbrough, used with permission.

Wherever you are
love is always there
in the sky watching
you until you do
something good
and when you do it
the love will come out of
    the sky
and come into you. Lily Johnson[10]

K-drama has deepened my appreciation of my granddaughter Lily's insight (Figure 2.3). Psychiatrist Chester Pierce taught us about the ways in which racism is enacted by micro-aggressions, very small acts that are barely noticeable.[11] Borrowing his concept to propose "micro-kindness," we see why K-drama slows down to show us a kindly smile, a courtesy, or a moment of acceptance.[12] Those small acts carry the moral code, enabling the major acts of sacrifice and transformation. They permit the traumatized to take chances.

In the eponymous show, the extraordinary attorney Wu's first day at work is animated by a lovely micro-kindness. She is on the autism spectrum and can't always interpret the world around her. She is befuddled by the building's revolving door and goes round and round helplessly. Lee Jun-ho, who works in the building, sees her struggling and stops to help. He shows her that by doing a waltz—1-2-3—she can dance her way out of the door and go home.

SmallGestures: Standing in the Face of Love

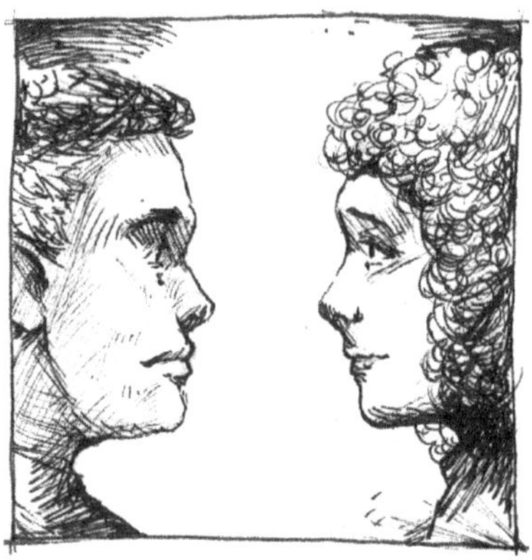

Figure 2.4 SmallGesture: Standing in the Face of Love.
Two people are looking at each other.
Drawing by Mike Malbrough, used with permission.

The K-drama *Business Proposal* was so silly that I feared the show wouldn't have a compelling lesson (Figure 2.4). Ha! The protagonist, Kang Tae-moo, had a childhood trauma: his parents were killed in a car crash during a rainstorm. He had posttraumatic stress disorder (PTSD), which was triggered by rain. His girlfriend, Shin Ha-ri, saw the symptoms of the PTSD when they got caught in the rain. Later, she learned about the cause. She used this knowledge to manage a subsequent storm, immediately covering him with a brilliant yellow umbrella once it started to rain. Then she said, "I have something I always wanted to do on a rainy-day date with a boyfriend, if I ever had a boyfriend."

That line is very disarming, because it focuses attention on her difficulties. She took him into the subway, which as a child of wealth he'd never ridden before, to a subway flower market, where he bought her an enormous bouquet, and to eat jeon, which she explained was the perfect food for that weather. By the time the rain had stopped and they were walking down the street, he had had an emotional breakthrough. He asked her, "How long have you known? I wanted to tell you, but I didn't want to look pathetic in front of the woman I love."

Father Richard Rohr compared such healings to the exorcisms performed by Jesus:

> In that sense, I've personally known a lot of possessed people. It's no surprise that Jesus exorcised so many demons from people who seemed to carry the negative projections of the surrounding crowd (Luke 9:37–43), synagogue worshippers (Mark 1:21–27; Luke 13:10–17), or the Gerasene residents (Mark 5:1–20; Luke 8:26–39). The ancients were not as naive as we might think. In these stories, we see exactly what the internalization of negative judgment means. Such people do need healing, even a major "exorcism"! While we tend to send them to therapists instead of holy people, in general, the only cure for negative possession is a positive repossession! Jesus is always "repossessing" people—for themselves and for God.
>
> When a good therapist, a wise and holy (meaning whole or healed) person, or a totally accepting friend becomes our chosen mirror, we are, in fact, being healed! I hope it doesn't sound too presumptuous, but I think I have exorcised a good number of people in my life—primarily because *they* had the trust and the humility to let me mirror them *positively* and replace the old mirror of their abusive dad, their toxic church, or their racist neighborhood. That's why Jesus says, "*Your* faith has saved you" (Luke 7:50). I am just saying the same.[13]

Shin Ha-ri is the totally accepting friend who mirrors acceptance to Kang Tae-moo, exorcising the demon of negative judgment that was keeping him from having peace. His faith in her permits him to give himself to her care on the rainy-day date. His faith saves him, enabling him to work through the family prejudice against Shin Ha-ri's working-class origins.

SmallGestures: Do the Next Right Thing

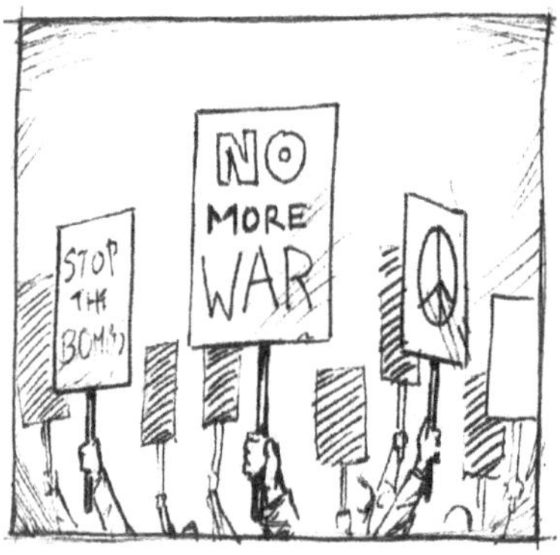

Figure 2.5 SmallGesture: Do the Next Right Thing.
People are demonstrating against war.
Drawing by Mike Malbrough, used with permission.

I have been a peace activist since I was a preteen demonstrating against atomic bombs (Figure 2.5). The first significant moral decision I ever made was to leave my candy striper training, which I thought would help me prepare to be a physician, to join a "Ban the Bomb" walk that went through New Jersey to New York City.[14]

In the 1960s that commitment to peace segued into the struggle to end the war in Vietnam. When I was a freshman at Bryn Mawr, I saw a petition on a bulletin board in Taylor Hall asking for signatures in support of men resisting the draft. Not only was resisting the draft illegal, but also supporting those who resisted carried the threat of penalties. I wanted to sign but was afraid, and my fear wrestled with my conscience. I was there for some time before I picked up my pen, thereby becoming a "Resister's Sister."

The stories of K-drama turn on this struggle. Because psychiatrist and anthropologist Dr. Arthur Kleinman is the leading thinker on the connection between moral crisis and illness, I pulled his books off the shelf.[15] One of the inspirations for his work was Dr. W. H. R. Rivers, a polymath who made major contributions in anthropology, physiology, and psychiatry. During World War I each of these parts of his background became important to the treatment of men with "shell shock." He had a unique insight into the suffering of his patients and was able to offer an "ethnographically informed" treatment. This meant that the world of the sufferer—before and during the war—was placed in conversation with the pain of the person. The officers he was treating were upper-class young men, raised to serve "God and country" with unflagging loyalty. Desertion was morally repugnant, but the war they were sent to fight was a death machine. The army was trapped in trenches and from time to time ordered to charge German lines—the trenches were deadly in one way, the charges in another. The officers, Dr. Rivers believed, broke under the strain of being caught between principle and near-certain death.

Dr. Kleinman explained how Dr. Rivers used the tools of ethnography and psychiatry in treating these men:

> The army officers Rivers treated were, he believed, experiencing neurotic symptoms because of conflicts between inner feelings, largely unconscious, of self-preservation and societal and military values that required them to be brave and steadfast in the trenches, where they could neither fall nor fight but had to passively persevere under shelling that appeared to kill soldiers randomly and over which they could exert no control at all—a terrifying reality. Seen this way, the conflicting moral worlds of his officer patients—their homes, schools, and the military

combat conditions they endured—were the sources of their illnesses. *Theirs were moral disorders.*[16]

Much of this approach is illustrated in Rivers's work with the famous poet Siegfried Sassoon, who had been sent to Craiglockhart War Hospital because he had taken a public stand against the war. When he asked Dr. Rivers if he had war neurosis, Dr. Rivers replied that he had an "anti-war complex." At the heart of Sassoon's dilemma was a moral choice: he could sit out the war in the hospital or he could go back, possibly to his death. To make such a choice, Dr. Rivers believed, Sassoon would have to face his moral dilemma.

The story of this famous doctor/patient encounter has been told in the novel and eponymous film *Regeneration*.[17] In the film, Dr. Rivers asks Sassoon how he would feel, being safe in Scotland, while others were in the trenches?

Another patient at the hospital at that time, Wilfred Owen, wrote a scathing poem attacking the code of their upper-class culture. He describes watching a man die from a gas attack and then says that had his listener seen all the horrors of that,

My friend, you would not tell with such high zest
To children ardent for some desperate glory,
The old Lie: *Dulce et decorum est*
Pro patria mori.[18]

I think both men were cured of their moral disorders. They came to terms with the choice they had to make. For both, a time at Craiglockhart, with its many small kindnesses, enabled them to come face to face with the love of Dr. Rivers and then to step into the harsh destiny that awaited them.[19] Sassoon went back to the war and received a head wound and was repatriated home. Owen went back to the war and was killed.

SmallGestures: The Party

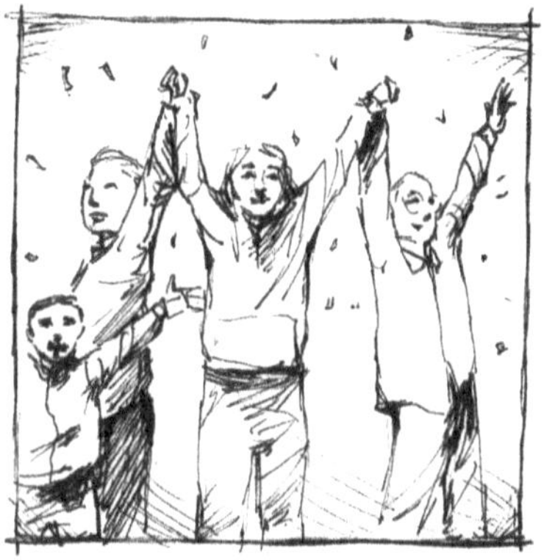

Figure 2.6 SmallGesture: The Party. People are celebrating.
Drawing by Mike Malbrough, used with permission.

There are joyous parties at the end of many K-dramas (Figure 2.6). At the end of *Our Blues*, the peer group that had struggled with crisis is practicing for some gathering. They want to assert the pride of their community over their rivals. As a viewer, I didn't know what was coming and laughed out loud as the competitions unfurled. I was almost hysterical with laughter by the time they started a kind of bumper-car contest in which people hopped on one leg to take out their opponent.

Often at the end of a show we see photos of the process of making the show and even a group shot of all the people involved in acting, makeup, costume, film, and sound. These group shots show glorious moments of joy, the very meta moment of reflecting the story's party with a party in real life.

SmallGestures serve as connectors for the fabric of collective life. Bill Morrish helped me see this web of relations. He took his drawing of the "Yin-Yang in the Narrative Arc of K-drama" (Figure 2.1) and repeated it many times, in all directions, to demonstrate the webs of connection and their pivot around the HeartMind—that is, where the SmallGestures that move the Chi are acting (Figure 2.7).[20]

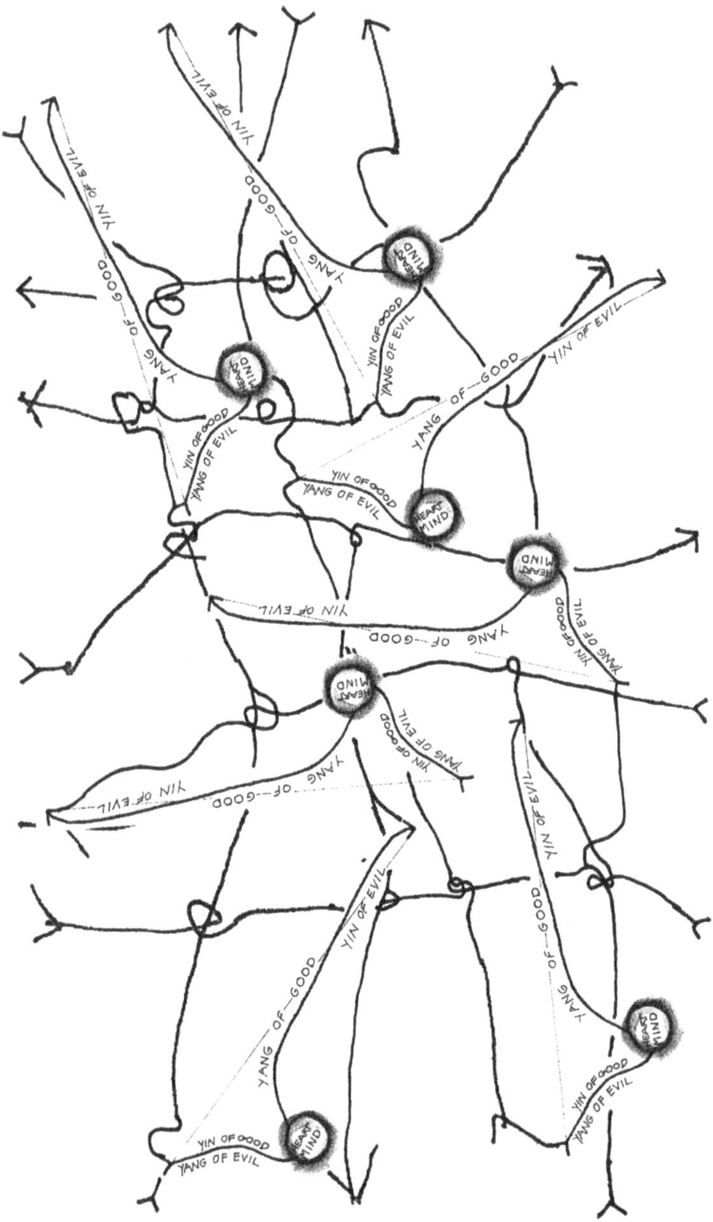

Figure 2.7 The Web of Stories.
This diagram shows multiple copies of the arc of yin/yang, connecting around the HeartMind to permit change.
Drawing by William Morrish, used with permission.

With Shamanism as the Foundation

One day Professor Rhonda Hughes, a K-drama-ophile I'd met through the lectures at Bryn Mawr, emailed me to say, "You have to watch *Dr. Romantic*."

I thought the title was a bit weird, but I followed her advice. I was immediately swept into the world of medicine and, in particular, all the moral crises that face physicians. I was profoundly shaken by the show. I needed to talk to someone, and I thought musician and writer Jun Bum Sun would be able to help. I was reaching out not with a precise question but rather with a *cri de coeur*—what was I feeling and why?

This took the conversation into Shamanism. He said, "Buddhism, Taoism, Confucianism, and Christianity are the superstructure of Korean thought, but the substructure is Shamanism."

The first thing non-Korean viewers—including me—come to know about K-drama is that it's fabulous. I mean that in every sense of the word—it is really great, really over-the-top stylish, really amazing. This is often dismissed as frivolous, but actually it is part of the deep wisdom the shows draw from Shamanism, the indigenous religion of the Korean peninsula that goes back thousands of years.

Shamanism sees our world as intertwined with the spirit world. Shamans are in touch with the spirit world, often themselves embodying a spirit familiar. Historically, shamans did their healing by gathering the collective for some days of storytelling, using the pattern language to tell stories that mirrored the issues their listeners were experiencing. In *Poong: Joseon Psychiatrist*, Dr. Poong gathers the community to tell a story that saves a woman at risk from bullying.[21] In just that way, shamans would invite a community to assemble for storytelling carried out by the whole gathering, with the community singing and dancing together. And it took time—often days. The 12 to 24 hours of a K-drama, with its painful beginning, difficult resolution, and joyful, albeit inconclusive, ending, are in the spirit of the shamans' tradition.

In addition to singing, dancing, and storytelling, Shamanism emphasized beauty—wearing makeup, dressing up, and looking fabulous. This suggests to me that the stylishness of K-drama—and Korean culture—has deep, deep roots in the peninsula's history.

The influence of Shamanism is also evident in K-drama's use of magical realism, a style of storytelling that has one foot in the mundane world we all recognize and the other foot in fantastical and mystical worlds. Things are never simply in one place, one time, one dimension. However many dimensions the shows draw on, we know there are more—past lives, future lives, other parallel worlds. As viewers, we find things familiar enough to enter the story yet unfamiliar enough to release us from our familiar patterns and expectations. This estrangement makes change possible, even inevitable.

The writers of K-drama, Jun Bum Sun proposed, are shaman adjacent, having some of the insight and perceptions of shamans. It is that ability to read between the lines, to perceive the deep conflicts, and to understand and respond to the archetypal patterns that informs their work and allows it to land so precisely.

I was comforted by my conversation with Jun Bum Sun, and I was consoled by *Dr. Romantic*. In particular, I had a completely different understanding of what had happened to me during my professional formation. While trying to be a good doctor, I made unethical, stupid, or ill-informed mistakes and my mentors scolded me for them. I felt deep shame about those acts and have held on to that shame all this time. *Dr. Romantic* showed me a host of physicians, at different stages in their careers, making exactly those kinds of errors and getting chewed out by Kim Sabu, Dr. Romantic himself. I saw something I'd never understood: that mistakes were part of the Path, and that scolding was part of the love mentors have for the younger people in their care. The process of change gives us the courage to be seen, to be scolded, to be healed, and in that way to return to the world as one of the helpful people, bending the arc of the moral universe toward justice.

This echoed a conversation I had had with Dr. Kong Jeong-ok and her husband Joe DiGangi while I was in Korea. Dr. Kong emphasized that Koreans love stories and grow up surrounded by the remarkable stories of Joseon, collected in the "Veritable Records of the Joseon Dynasty." These stories were created by historians who wrote down everything the kings did—and the kings were forbidden to read what they wrote. There are hundreds of books of the Veritable Records, she told me, and people love to read them. There are even children's versions. K-drama takes these stories and uses them to hold a mirror up to society.

Part of K-drama's precision in drawing characters and understanding trauma is that families have been through so much that is in living memory. Dr. Kong's grandmother grew up during a time when Korea was a Japanese colony. Her grandmother married at age 16, as many people rushed daughters into marriage to protect them from sex slavery. Her parents grew up just before the Korean War, and her father remembered the war. When her mother was three or four, she was almost left behind by her parents as they tried to escape their village. They thought she might be dead. This story was "calmly" related to Dr. Kong, who told me, "The people writing K-dramas are the children and grandchildren of the people who survived Japanese colonization, the Korean War, and the building of capitalism. They have heard the stories and saw what happened to people's lives—they are bringing all of our history to the screen."

We talked at length about *My Liberation Notes*, and they put the whole show into perspective for me.[22] I live an hour and a half from New York City, and it is not a wasteland. This colored my perception of the travails of the three siblings in the show who live in the countryside and commute to work in Seoul. Dr. Kong and Joe DiGangi were emphatic that I had the wrong model. The villages had been emptied out as the young people moved to Seoul to find work. Later during my time in Korea I visited artist Lee Kyungho at his studio. He explained that he'd lived in such a rural place for a year and showed me a video he'd made of a bus stop on a nearly empty road. It could have been location research for *My Liberation Notes.*

I try to watch carefully, to read about the shows, and to speak to people who are Korean or Korean American. Grace Jang, in her book *K-drama School,* notes that the Korean War is in her body. I did not grow up in that aspect of the Cold War, which was waged between capitalism and communism in the 1950s—instead, I grew up in the Cold War against labor, which split my father's union and cost him both his job and the civil rights organization he had built.[23] These experiences are not separate, but they are not the same. This requires that I keep growing in my openness to stories from a different country with a different culture. Everything that follows reflects the imperfections and wonder inherent in such a project.

Yet there comes a time in a project such as this when one must take a stand. I have proposed that there is a "Tao of K-drama"—and at this point I must say what I think it is. One of the diagrams I drew in the course of this work is shown in Figure 2.8—16 tumbling triangles, standing for change in each of the 16 episodes of a show.

K-drama asks: how do we ride these waves? The Tao of K-drama teaches that the injured self can be healed and can rejoin the collective. The Tao of K-drama emphasizes that we are not healing the self solely for the self but to become "*oori*"—Korean for "we the family of us"—so that we are all riding the waves, searching for the keys to be a collective, held together by love in spite of precarity,

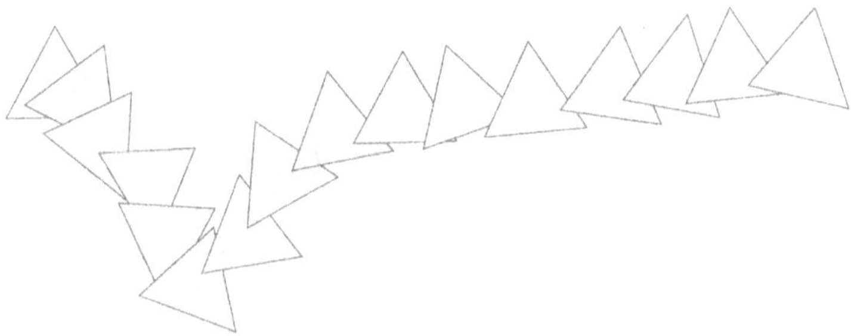

Figure 2.8 Dancing Triangles.
There are 16 episodes in a K-drama and in this diagram there are 16 triangles, symbolizing the integrity of each episode, with its own ups and downs and tasks, as well as the episode's situation within the narrative arc of the show.

and buoyed by joy. In K-drama we see that as *oori*, we can help to make a change in the world.

In the next seven chapters I will examine seven of the 88 K-dramas that inform this proposition.

3

Peace in the Heart

Heo Im Gets Sent to the School of Hard Knocks

Hard knocks is a rough school, but a fool will learn in no other.

—African American folk saying

"I can't believe that great doctor was such a brat."

—Dr. Choi Chun-sool, *Live Up to Your Name, Dr. Heo!*

One who makes promises lightly is sure to have little credibility;
One who finds everything easy is certain to have lots of difficulties.

—*The Tao*, No. 63

I studied acupuncture with Dr. Michael O. Smith at Lincoln Recovery Center in the South Bronx in the early 1980s. For those who know about "Lincoln Acupuncture," as it was fondly called, that sentence will bring back so many memories: the wildness of the South Bronx, which had been decimated by the brutal anti-urban policy of "planned shrinkage"; the low building facing a small park and its wide doors that welcomed people in; the big treatment room with its comfortable armchairs; the team of acupuncturists circulating to give ear acupuncture to anyone who came in; and the fact that all you had to do to get that acupuncture was sit in a chair.

Mike was an extraordinary doctor. When I met him, I was a fourth-year resident in psychiatry with three young children at home. I was very tired all the time. He would give me acupuncture while teaching me about how it worked. I would invariably fall asleep. "Don't worry," he would say, "the information gets in."

There is a photo of Mike sitting at his desk in front of his packed bookcase, looking over his glasses at someone who is out of the shot. I sat there many times while Mike explained his view of the body and its treatment. He too was a psychiatrist, so we shared a reverence for the life of the mind. At the heart of addiction is the loss of control over one's mind and actions. He taught me that the goal of treatment was to create a space in which the person might begin to make decisions again: "A person could sit on the bench in the park outside and decide to be sober. It is the work of a moment. The acupuncture quiets the craving enough that the person can have that moment."

I loved Mike, and I loved acupuncture. And so when Netflix offered me *Live Up to Your Name,* a Korean show about an acupuncturist, I clicked on it. *Live Up to Your Name* is the story of Heo Im, who must resolve his resentments and grudges if he is to become the great doctor he is destined to be. To help him along this path, he gets a dose of the future.

> The show opens by a river. It is obviously the olden days, and various people are sharpening tools on stones by the water. Among them is a man who is sharpening a set of acupuncture needles. His assistant comes by to tell him to wash up and come to work. She runs off, moving through the courtyard of a massive place, calling, "Everyone, everyone, let's start!'
>
> Her joy is infectious, and the music shifts, gathering speed and delight. She runs and opens massive doors. "Come in!" she calls to the crowd of people gathered there.

If Lincoln Recovery Center had had a soundtrack, it would have been rap, of course, because it was the South Bronx in the 1980s. But it would have had the same joy, which in part comes from the acupuncture itself, as Mike taught it, a treatment that calms us and opens us to our own best ideas.

How could I not love *Live Up to Your Name*?

Chutes and Ladders

Like Siegfried Sassoon and Wilfred Owen, Heo Im is caught between his suffering and his moral obligations. Sassoon and Owen were enabled to recover through treatment at Craiglockhart War Hospital. Heo Im does not receive "treatment" in that sense. Rather, as the older doctor, Heo Jun, supposed, Heo Im had been through a lot. His ups and downs reminded me of the ancient Indian spiritual game Snakes and Ladders. We know this game as Chutes and Ladders, a simple board game in which one advances on a roll of the dice. If you land on a chute, you slide backward. If you land on a ladder, you jump forward.

I made symbols for ladders and chutes and went through the show again. While I had documented what happened in the show, the resulting diagram did not reveal the "how": how did Heo Im become enlightened? I reworked the diagram with a simpler concept: did the act lead to hope or despair? And that worked—even the first crude draft showed me pieces I'd been missing, the intricate dance of negative and positive feedback that drives Heo Im's thinking in the direction of understanding what Heo Jun refers to as "the meaning and value of your skills" to help reveal the "how."

Near the end of the show, we can see that service in the Imjin War did not make Heo Im happy. He was, however, able to endure the hardship, and that, many would say, is the goal of spiritual practice: the ability to manage what life throws at us. I was also able to see the steps through which he transformed from brat to partner and the several ways in which the teachings arrived.

How does this get put together?

When I was growing up in Orange, New Jersey, in the 1950s, "tack head" was the expression used for people who wouldn't listen to their elders or do the right thing. It was a derogatory way of saying that they were hard-headed and disrespectful. They were condemned to learn in the "School of Hard Knocks."

Heo Im is certainly such a person. Though we understand the trauma that has driven him in that direction, the question of how to break through to him is a major one. That's where the Great Powers' extreme intervention of time travel comes in. By lifting Heo Im out of Joseon, needle case in hand, the Great Powers have put him in a situation where he has to make choices, each of which will have consequences. And that feedback loop is what will get through to him. In my family therapy training, my supervisors said we had to "pat and kick" to get families to change. We were to start with a "pat" of encouragement and follow that with a "kick" of criticism. In Heo Im's School of Hard Knocks these are experienced as "chutes," painful setbacks (downward spirals), and "ladders," experiences that reinforce his good deeds (upward arrows).

Heo Im's Journey

There was a real man, Heo Im, who is known as one of the greatest acupuncturists in Korean history.[1] But in the show we meet a gifted man who is unable to be promoted because of his class origins. His work in a public clinic prohibits him from treating the rich, but he sneaks out at night to do so. He can't spend his gold, so he has piled it up and dances with his gold and riches at night. Filled with resentment because of his situation, Heo Im goes mad with greed and abandons good medical sense. When called to treat the king, Heo Im abandons Yeon-i, a poor girl with an illness only he can cure, to rush to the palace. I have included excerpts from my timeline, accompanied by drawings by Mike Malbrough, to illustrate Heo Im's journey of restoration (Figure 3.1).

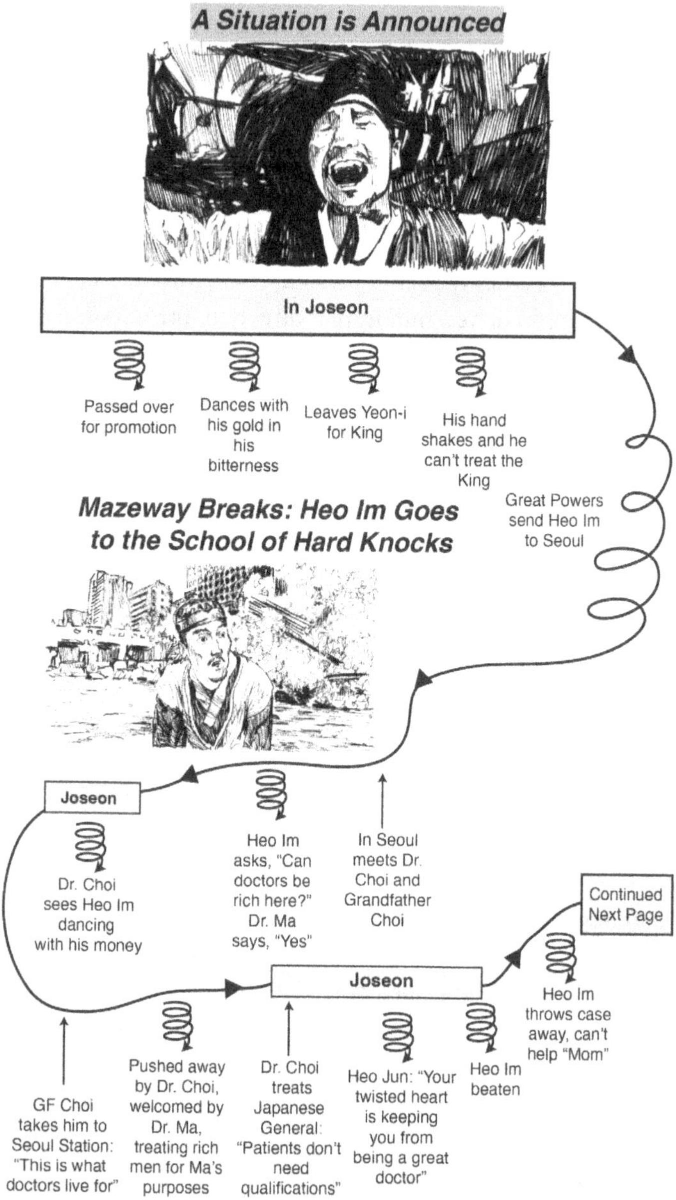

Figure 3.1 Heo Im's Journey of Restoration.
Mike Malbrough took the concept of "Chutes and Ladders" to lay out the timeline of Heo Im's journey through the six stages of the Arc of Restoration. The "chutes" are downward spirals and the "ladders" are upward-pointing arrows.
Drawings and design by Mike Malbrough, used with permission.

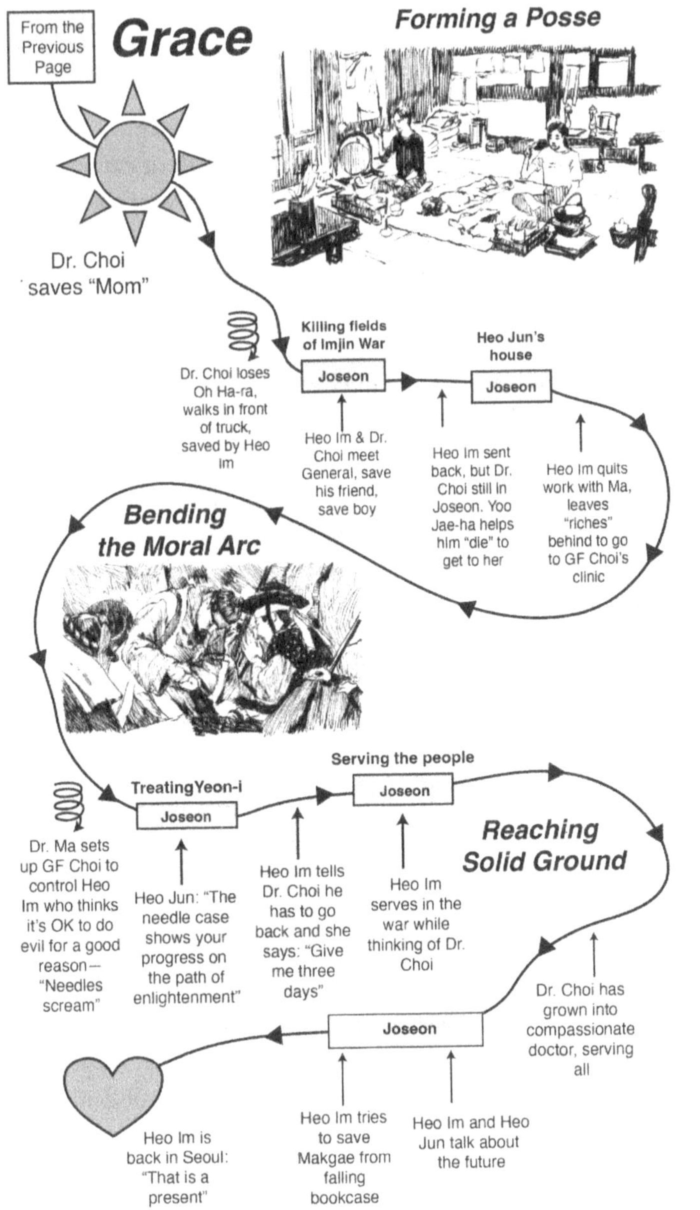

Figure 3.1 Continued

Heo Im's abandonment of Yeon-i is too much for the Powers-of-the-Universe. As happens in many magical stories, the Great Powers send Heo Im on a journey. In the Western canon, such a story often involves an "old crone" sitting by a creek who asks a handsome young man if he would carry her across. He looks at her with disgust and says, "Why would I do that?" She then reveals who she really is and sends him on a journey to learn how to behave.

In Heo Im's case, in the presence of the king, his hand shakes and he is unable to carry out the treatment. He is then sent to the 21st century carrying a magic needle box (Figure 3.1). He lands in a river and is stunned by the modern world—this is the breaking of the mazeway of his everyday life, opening him to new questions and new answers. There he meets famed acupuncturist Choi Chun-sool. While watching the time-traveling Heo Im, Dr. Choi shakes his head and says, "I can't believe that great doctor was such a brat."

Moral Choice and Trauma

There is an important connection between moral choice and trauma. The kinds of trauma that produce mental illness are those that threaten a person's life. In the aftermath of such experiences, people reason—often unconsciously—"I am at risk so I need to take care of myself, not trust others to do it." This becomes elaborated in what Bill Wilson, cofounder of Alcoholics Anonymous, called "self-centered fear," which basically means "my needs trump yours."[2] This is a fraught position because self-centered fear is always in tension with morality, and this creates a secondary problem for the self: self-preservation battles with the self-esteem that comes from doing right. The traumatized person is in a no-win situation: To be alive but ashamed? To be proud but dead?

When Heo Im arrives in modern Seoul, his first question is "Can doctors be rich here?" This reveals his priorities, and clearly, he's in major trouble. He sees a magnificent Oriental medicine hospital as the answer to his prayers. Of course—because he asked the wrong question—he encounters the avatar of greed, the ambitious Dr. Ma, who will open a chute for him!

> When Dr. Ma had met Heo Jun, Heo Im's older colleague, 20 years earlier he'd tried to use him for his selfish purposes but Heo Jun had scruples and rebuffed him. Now Dr. Ma wishes to use Heo Im, recently arrived from Joseon, for his evil machinations.
>
> But the Great Powers are looking out for Heo Im. They place him in the path of the traumatized surgeon, Choi Yeon-kyung, his equal in talent for healing. When they first meet, he annoys her and is taken off to the police station. By "chance," he encounters Choi Yeon-kyung's grandfather, Dr. Choi Chun-sool. Grandfather Choi recognizes that the disheveled time traveler is the great acupuncturist Heo Im.
>
> Heo Im spends the night at Grandfather Choi's house, which is a traditional Seoul hanok house, built around a courtyard where there is a large platform, the *jangdokdae.* In the morning, the older women of the neighborhood gather in the courtyard. Grandfather Choi treats them right there on the jangdokdae, adding to his gentle touch wise thoughts about the ways in which our bodies carry all we have learned from life.
>
> One of the women patients, who has begun to lose her memory, carries a small pet pig, which she thinks of as her son. She asks Heo Im to treat the pig. He is a little shocked but does as she asks. When the pig is better, Heo Im smiles—he is always delighted when the ill are healed. Grandfather Choi sees this, and he understands how to help the time traveler. Meanwhile, the old lady transfers her affection from the pig to Heo Im. She thinks of him as her long-lost son and he starts to think of her as "Mom."

There is much joy in this meeting at Grandfather Choi's clinic, and I recognized in that morning of laughter and hope the same deep healing that so many of us received at Lincoln Recovery

Center. Mike Smith often told me that, if properly tuned, the healing energy emanating from each of our bodies filled the whole room; just being in the room helped a person feel better. Heo Im is severely out of balance, but the power of that morning marks the beginning of healing for him. I speculate that this scene of gathering, care, and joy is analogous to the Shamanistic healing rituals in which the community gathers for singing and dancing to heal the wounded souls, including their collective soul.

> Later, Grandfather Choi takes Heo Im to Seoul Station where homeless men are squatting. Heo Im delivers the first of many remarkable treatments, saving the life of a man who has water intoxication. Grandfather Choi comments that helping people is what gives doctors joy.
>
> Twenty years earlier Grandfather Choi had encountered another time traveler, Heo Jun, also a master of Oriental medicine. Like most masters, Heo Jun has had his own troubles, which were so severe at one point that he was unable to practice medicine. At that time, the Great Powers sent Heo Jun to Seoul with the needle case. He met the troubled family of Grandfather Choi. He stabilized Grandfather Choi's granddaughter, Dr. Choi Yeon-kyung, who had just witnessed the death of her father, Grandfather Choi's son. Both by caring for his granddaughter and by setting an example of taking the right path in spite of its costs, Heo Jun gave Grandfather Choi courage to live a moral life.
>
> Meanwhile, the evil Dr. Ma is there to entice Heo Im over to the dark side. Dr. Ma wants to use Heo Im's unmatched skills to win the support of rich and influential men for his own ends. He gets Heo Im a fraudulent license and welcomes him into the Oriental medicine hospital. There, Heo Im thinks he has it made, but he celebrates too soon. Time after time, Dr. Ma calls him to make "house calls" to famous men who have something to hide. At first, Heo Im is excited to show off his skill, but that wears off

quickly and he is left disgusted by the arrogance and duplicity of the wealthy. He finds that the wealthy in modern Seoul are just as disgusting as the wealthy in Joseon.

In one episode, he is taken to treat the addicted son of a wealthy man who wants to hide his son's addiction. The son escapes the house but collapses in the street. At the hospital, Dr. Choi Yeon-kyung finds he has a heart valve infection and wants to treat him. The father, terrified the secret of his son's addiction will get out, sends his thugs and Heo Im to get his son back from the hospital. Choi Yeon-kyung fights to keep him in her care, but Heo Im humiliates her to get control of the situation.

The machinations of Dr. Ma invite Heo Im to enact evil while the humble invitations of Grandfather Choi engage him in good works—these represent the "chutes" and "ladders." He is also dragged back and forth in time, "knocks" that are disorienting and confusing. He is reminded over and over about the moral path of a doctor, which becomes his lifeline for finding his way. The rapid-fire series of experiences begins to build in his Heart-Mind as we move toward the turning point (Figure 3.1).

Episode 10, I find, is often a pivotal moment in K-drama. In this show, that is when the conflict between the paths comes to a head. Here's the way in which the pivot plays out in *Live Up to Your Name*:

In Joseon, the servant Du Chil begs Heo Im to treat his brother, also a servant, without the master's permission. The master finds out and has the brother killed. Heo Im debases himself to plead for Du Chil and himself. He knows that Choi Yeon-Kyeong has seen his humiliation. When Heo Im returns to Seoul, he throws the needle case away and spurns the homeless people who ask for his help. But no sooner has he turned away from the Path than he finds his "Mom" passed out on the street. He reaches for his needle case, but it is not there. He screams for help and sobs in despair. This is the ultimate chute.

Dr. Choi Yeon-kyung arrives and saves "Mom." And that is the ultimate ladder, the moment of grace. This is a definitive moment for Heo Im, who turns away from greed and toward the moral path (Figure 3.1).

Dr. Choi Yeon-kyung, however, has her own problems related to the tragic death of her father, which she has repressed. When she loses a special patient, she goes through her own crisis. She and Heo Im are sent back to Joseon, and there they must work together to save a boy who has been shot by a Japanese soldier. This is the point at which Heo Im begins to form the posse with whom he will work to put new patterns on the world (Figure 3.1).

Dr. Ma, of course, does not want to let go of the Golden Goose and seeks to control Heo Im by framing Grandfather Dr. Choi, a move that had failed when he'd tried to use it on Heo Jun. Dr. Choi, his granddaughter Dr. Choi Yeon-kyung, the homeless people, and Heo Im have to work together to solve the crisis Dr. Ma creates. This leads Heo Im to a deeper understanding of the full meaning and power of "doing good."

Faced with his new knowledge, he returns to Joseon, intending to treat Yeon-i, the girl whose abandonment triggered his ejection into the future. Once that task is complete, he plans to return to Seoul. But what he has been learning will change his path.

There is an important conversation between Heo Im and his mentor Heo Jun that happens during this visit to Joseon.

Heo Im is sitting near Heo Jun, who is brewing herbs for his patients.[3] Heo Im pulls out the needle case. He looks at the case and then at Heo Jun and says, "I heard this belonged to you."

"That is not mine," Heo Jun responds. "That stayed with me temporarily. As to how long that needle box has existed and how long it stays in someone's hands, I do not know all the secrets.

I only know I had the chance to become a doctor again thanks to that box and that I eventually came back here. I think it wants to protect. That is my guess."

"Protect?"

"Doctors are rare at this time. More so for extraordinary doctors. There must be a reason that needle box chose you, especially when we are at war. If my guess is right, you must know the meaning and value of your skills. You said you would not take any memories from here with you, but you returned on your own to save a child at this dangerous time. The box's choice was not wrong."

Heo Im looks at the box intently. "What are these patterns?"

"You must have been through a lot. It signifies the enlightenment you found and the progress of your change as a doctor."

"I have not seen this before."

"It must be time," Heo Jun opines, meaning the end of the journey that Heo Im has been on, traveling back and forth in time, and moving from resentment to acceptance, even love.

He returns to Seoul with a heavy heart, finally clear that his gift is meant to be put at the service of the people of Joseon who have no one else. Heo Im and Dr. Choi Yeon-kyung say a tearful goodbye, knowing what duty calls them each to do: that is their enlightenment.

The Needle Box Wants to Protect

In the Western version of this story, the journey is certainly a punishment for not being willing to help the weak. In this show, I had thought of the time travel as punishment for choosing greed over service.

By contrast, Heo Jun puts forward the idea that the Great Powers want to protect—I was surprised when Heo Jun said that. "Who or what is to be protected?" I wondered. That became clear when Heo Jun observes that "Doctors are rare." Therefore, the Great Powers are protecting *the people* by restoring their doctors, and especially their most gifted doctors, to their work.

In the show, we saw the Joseon-era public clinic where Heo Im worked thronged with dozens of poor people, thrilled to be waiting for the great doctor and confident he can make them well. Many explained they'd traveled great distances to see him. Their need was desperate. Instead of being grateful that he could be of service, Heo Im was disdainful and preoccupied with his own resentments. He could and did abandon the people, because his values were out of whack. The Great Powers needed to protect the people—all those people who had little hope if it were not for Heo Im.

> We watch Heo Im's service in the Imjin War, suffering through terrible cold and dodging blows to deliver care to the wounded, all the time grieving that he will never see Choi Yeon-kyung again (Figure 3.1).
>
> After the war, he is called to treat the king for tinnitus, that annoying ringing in the ears that won't go away. On his way to the king, Heo Im encounters a wounded boy. He sends the servant to tell the king that he has to care for his subject first.
>
> He remembers the king and the court abandoning the people during the war and wonders if the tinnitus, known in Oriental medicine as the "cry of the heart," is remorse for leaving. He treats the king for that, and it is successful. He is—finally—offered a position as a physician to the king.
>
> Later, talking with Heo Jun, he complains that his service in the war was not recognized, but this trivial treatment of the king brings reward. Heo Jun, ever the master, replies, "Rewards are not for meaningless things, but sometimes you get something you didn't expect—that is a present."

Then they argue about who's more famous in the 21st century, which is pretty funny. But most important, we see that Heo Im has learned that enlightenment is seeing past one's own greed and wish for comfort so that one can make the right choice. Enlightenment does not mean that you get the "happy ending." The terrible scenes on the battlefield, dreaming of Choi Yeon-kyung with no way to see her again, are testament to Heo Im's evolution as a person, able to be of service to his society in spite of his personal suffering.

Heo Im started off asking, "Can doctors get rich here?" but he learned to ask the better question: "Can I join in helping others?"

That would seem to be the end, but there are two surprises in the Cracker Jack box of this show.

> The first is that Dr. Ma, disgraced and dismissed, also finds the moral path. What a surprise when he shows up at Dr. Choi's clinic with containers of food wrapped in cloth. He invites Dr. Choi to have lunch with him. Sitting on the platform, Dr. Ma explains, "Since I gave up greed and my bad reputation, like you said, my heart and body are healthier than ever."
>
> He asks for a job, but Dr. Choi scoffs, "It's a poor clinic." Then Dr. Ma offers to work for free. The men laugh and Dr. Choi accepts.

My friend Dr. Marisela Gomez, a Buddhist in the tradition of Thich Naht Hanh, loves that teaching about greed and often refers to it when we talk about K-drama.

> The second surprise is that Heo Im gets caught by a falling bookcase and time travels again to Seoul. Choi Yeon-kyung wants to know how long he's staying. He says, "I've come to live with you—I couldn't live without you any longer."
>
> We watch them walk off into the sunset surrounded by a heart. Can he really stay? We don't know (Figure 3.1).

What Is Solid Ground?

The last part of the arc of restoration is "reaching solid ground." I don't view Heo Im's surprise visit to Seoul at the end as "solid ground." Maybe the key here is that I invented the category "solid ground"; K-drama didn't. Maybe it represents my Western ideal of "closure"—settled, done. As Sergeant Preston of the Yukon would say to his beautiful dog, "Well, King, I guess this case is closed."

K-dramas don't close so much as end. And viewers who like a Western ending constantly ask Google, "Is there a season 2 of___?" because in season 2, we get closure.

Should I, therefore, abandon "reaching solid ground" as the final stage of the arc of restoration?

If "solid" means "happily ever after," I should.

But I've learned a new meaning of "solid," the one spiritual teachers—including my own—are always trying to get across. That "solid" is something inside us that allows us to achieve and hold a moral posture. This is like ballet, which trains the muscles to hold us upright, even on our tiptoes. In the K-drama *Navillera*, Shim Deok-chul is desperate to learn ballet, but he has encroaching Alzheimer's. Despite his advancing illness, his young teacher Lee Chae-rok is confident that he can perform in a show because he has muscle memory of the dance. And so it proves. A year after the show, he encounters his teacher, who had been struggling to achieve stardom in the dance world. Through the dense fog of his memory loss, he remembers the young man and asks, "Did you soar?"[4]

If, in life or through K-drama, we have learned what we were supposed to learn, it will keep us steady—and that is the solid ground for which we are striving; it is what allows us to soar.

We come out from behind our greed and fear to do the next right thing.

4

Peace in the Home

Cha Eun-ho Gets a Roommate

. . . let that page come out of you—
Then, it will be true.
I wonder if it's that simple?
—Langston Hughes, *Theme for English B*

"I smell a best-seller."
—President Kim Tae-woo, *Romance Is a Bonus Book*

Way-making is so profuse as to be nameless (*wuming*).
It is only way-making that is as efficacious in the beginning of things
As it is in their completion.
—*The Tao*, No. 41

In Western fairytales, the marriage comes at the end and the couple lives happily ever after.

In the K-drama *Romance Is a Bonus Book,* the marriage occurs at the beginning and it's a flop.

We know it can't possibly work, because her husband-to-be isn't cute and he does a terrible, horrible, no-good, very bad dance down the aisle to the altar. Our suspicion is reinforced by the song that is playing. Called "Happy End," it has the telling line "Tell me now, *even lie*, that things will be all right."

When the marriage falls apart, as it must, Kang Dan-i is left supporting herself and their child. After 52 tries, she has not been able to get back into the marketing world, in which she excelled before she took a break from work to raise her daughter. She has part-time jobs at a sauna and a supermarket but cannot make ends meet. Her marital home is now abandoned and she has been sneaking into it at night. She wakes up to a wrecking ball thwacking the house. The demolition team looks at her with pity and horror as she stumbles away with her belongings. While rushing to a job interview that day, she loses her shoe. She is unemployed, homeless, and shoeless, and as if that were not enough, it starts to rain. Her best friend Cha Eun-ho calls and says, "Where are you?"

She replies, "I am at the edge of my life."

Kang Dan-i and Cha Eun-ho have a lot to sort out. He has to get her back from the edge; she has to find a way forward. Langston Hughes's poem, excerpted in the chapter epigraph, talks about a teacher's assignment to write what's inside you and it will be true.[1] Hughes asks what this show asks: is it that simple?

We don't know how complicated it will be, but because this is K-drama, we know it won't be simple for Kang Dan-i and Cha Eun-ho to find a way out of the friend zone. And in the process, they will need to untangle a succession of secrets, each of which is emblematic of the deep problem of precarity examined in the show.

The music in the show guides us through the intertwined themes. In one musical number, women of all sizes dance through Dan-i's workplaces as the song "Powerdance" pounds out these lyrics in English:

> When you're feeling like you're drowning . . .
> Get up now on your feet . . .
> 멋지게 Powerdance![2]

I wish I'd known that song when I was a medical student and resident and often had to tell myself to get up on my feet! To me, it felt like the segue from the bitterness of "Happy End" to the self-talk one tries in the face of deep despair.

Music is fundamental to Korean life, an inheritance from the Shamanistic beliefs and rituals Jun Bum Sun had told me about, and every K-drama has music. Sometimes the soundtrack will be composed of several strong ballads. Other times it will be oldies that support the storytelling, which is the case for *Prison Playbook*. And still other times it will be a full original score. *Romance Is a Bonus Book* has such a soundtrack, written by one of Korea's greatest composers, Nam Hye Seung. I asked filmmaker Billy Kent about the role of the soundtrack in the show. He described soundtracks as the voice of the director, sharing all that we can't see but need to know.

In particular, the music reveals the inner feelings of the characters. Dan-i's theme—"Powerdance"—contrasts with Eun-ho's theme, the tender ballad "All I Do." We might wonder about that message, and it will take a while for us to understand the secret he's carrying and why. Yet the placement of the music urges us to think about the contrast of the frenetic with the gently pleading. Composer Nam Hye-seung takes us, through the words and actions, into the painful secrets that our heroes hold.

Leaving the Friend Zone: The Story of Eun-ho and Dan-i's love

Eun-ho has known Dan-i since she saved his life when they were children. Though he has loved her for many years, he hadn't seen her in a while and didn't know her life had fallen apart. She is secretly working as his housekeeper, and since the demolition of her old house, secretly sleeping in his attic. On his kitchen counter she finds an advertisement for a job at his company. It is far below her skill level and would require that she conceal her excellent education and work achievements. We see her tear up symbols of

> all she has accomplished. Eun-ho has a profound shock when he walks into the interview room and sees Dan-i there. He demands to know what she's doing. She avoids answering. The company president loves her application and hires her, much to Eun-ho's dismay.
>
> Over the next few days, she is openly working at the publishing house, where Eun-ho has an important position. At night, she sneaks into his house. One evening he hears a strange noise and goes to investigate. Dan-i, moving around in the kitchen, hides. He turns out the light and pretends to go back to his room. Relieved, Dan-i comes out of hiding and that's when he catches her. He is shocked again.

This is a bold allusion to *Parasite*, the universally acclaimed 2019 K-film.[3] *Parasite* depicts a complicated and bizarrely intimate encounter between members of the poor Kim family and the affluent Park family. When the Parks go on vacation, their stunning contemporary mansion is occupied by the Kim family. The "squatters" begin uncovering the house's secrets, including the "ghost" in the basement who is revealed to be the husband of the Parks' former housekeeper. This revelation is among many symptoms of Korea's class divide. As the rich get richer, the poor might adopt parasitic behaviors, clinging to the wealthy for survival.

In *Romance Is a Bonus Book,* Dan-i has been turned down for 52 jobs. If that, plus her working part-time jobs, standing shoeless in the rain, and being willing to conceal her achievements to take a job far below her skill level, has not impressed us with the nature of things, the *Parasite* moment brings it home. Dan-i and Eun-ho have a "talk": she is hostile and embarrassed and hoping he'll let her stay. He is troubled and frightened for her. But she is his beloved, so of course she can stay. It will take a bit for his horror that "Dan-i's in *my* house?" to transform to joy that "*Dan-i's* in my house!" And it will take the whole show for it to transform to "*oori jib*," our house.

Work and Struggle

Kang Dan-i determined to find her way now that she has a chance, energetically performs the demeaning jobs she is assigned at the publishing house. She puts paper in the copier and calls for repairs. She makes lunch reservations. She refills the juice, coffee, and tea in the staff kitchen. She runs out to buy iced vanilla lattes for the executives' meeting. She packs up books. She even takes Associate Director Go Yu-seon's clothes to the dry cleaner.

She hopes to leverage up to the kind of work she's able to do. She gets a copy of an about-to-be-published book and works on writing a blurb for the cover. When rebuffed for her efforts, she doesn't give up. And she brings a sunny smile and deep affection for everyone to her work. Of course, Cha Eun-ho makes sure she has cute clothes and a stylish haircut. I mean, let's be real: she had no chance in her old black suit.

As things progress, Cha Eun-ho begins to woo Kang Dan-i. Their first outing involves an afternoon in Seoul. They listen to street musicians and enjoy the trio playing at a jazz bar. At another bar, Kang Dan-i wins at darts, to their great delight.

This is what I'm going to call the "Shaman's moment," the interlude when the energy shifts. It is different from the more gleeful "dating collage" we often see in shows when the couple goes bike riding together. This is a moment on the path to understanding. It shares with Grandfather Dr. Choi's clinic the warmth of gathering, this time in the public space. But Kang Dan-i is oblivious to Cha Eun-ho's feelings.

Though annoyed, Cha Eun-ho doesn't give up. He is helped by the arrival of a handwritten book, which has to be typed. The suggestion that Kang Dan-i perform this task is challenged by Dan-i's nemesis, Associate Director Go Yu-seon. "The book has a lot of Chinese characters," notes the associate director, assuming that "minimally educated" Kang Dan-i is not up to the task.

"I know a lot of Chinese characters," Kang Dan-i pipes up.

"Ohhhh, Kang Dan-i!" coo her coworkers in admiration of yet another of her talents.

And so Cha Eun-ho and Kang Dani-i are sent home to work. At one point, she rests her head on his shoulder, seeming to be asleep. He caresses her nose and mouth with his finger. When she gets up, she wonders what that feeling was and runs a pencil over her face to see if that is what she felt (Figure 4.1).

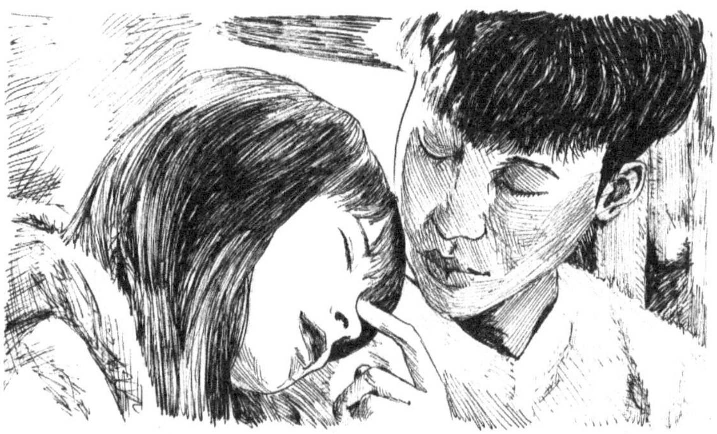

Figure 4.1 Kang Dan-i and Cha Eun-ho.
Cha Eun-ho traces Kang Dan-i's features as her head rests on his shoulder.
Drawing by Mike Malbrough, used with permission.

> Then snow starts to fall, the first snow of the season, held to be auspicious if couples experience it together. They go outside and Cha Eun-ho, by indirection, expresses his liking for her.

Kang Dan-i is a bit of what 1950s girls' books called "a romp"—a delightful character who doesn't take life too seriously. One could be a "sad romp"—a disparaging term—but Kang Dan-i is not that at all. She is just a bit untethered, which leads her to turn left when she should turn right. That is how she tumbled into a terrible marriage. But in that moment, when she finally intuits Cha Eun-ho's affection, she steps into reality.

> Cha Eun-ho begins to challenge her assumptions and fears. When she expresses her terror that by dating they might upset the apple cart of their precious relationship, he reassures her that they can be together forever. He helps her get to the truth that she adores him as much as he adores her. Once that is established, the tables turn, and Cha Eun-ho's secret, which was also hiding in the attic, is revealed. Once she knows the trouble he's carrying, Kang Dan-i can love him even more.

Back at the Office

Back at the office with the book perfectly typed, the K-drama works its way through a number of violence-laced office upheavals.

Workplaces in K-drama portray violence that is hard for me to witness. In *Twenty Five Twenty One*, the young reporter is kicked by his supervisor. In *Misaeng*, Jang Geu-rae is denied the protective clothing needed to check barrels of pickled squid. He is not informed when the task has finished and so continues his effort, ruining his good suit as a result. In *Romance Is a Bonus Book*, Song Hae-rin refuses to train a new employee whose attitude she finds to be too casual. When that woman makes a serious mistake,

Song Hae-rin shows her rage by thwacking her belt on a table in a terrifying manner. The violence moves outside the workplace too: Song Hae-rin's parents get angry at Cha Eun-ho because he doesn't like their daughter. One pushes him into a busy street, while the other trips him. They are then satisfied that they have taken their "revenge."

But physical violence and public humiliation are not the worst of it. Similar to *Parasite,* it is the violence of precarity that we are supposed to see and understand. Kang Dan-i has gotten her job by concealing her pedigree. When this is revealed, Associate Director Go Yu-seon, ready to seize any opportunity to get rid of Kang Dan-i, insists she resign. Cha Eun-ho says absolutely not, as it is not against the law to conceal one's credentials. But Kang Dan-i is quickly forced out and must again look for work.

Firing is a crisis for any individual, as well as others in their household.[4]

> By the time she is fired, Kang Dan-i and Cha Eun-ho are dating, so he wakes up early and makes her breakfast. She arrives at the table very upset. He points out the nice breakfast he has made for her. She is impressed by all the dishes and starts to feel better. Then he says he will do whichever of three things she would like: make a scene at the office, give her his credit card, or spend the day with her. She considers all the options and chooses "spend the day." They read, cuddle, and enjoy each other, which helps her get back on her feet.

To help Kang Dan-i with her job search, Cha Eun-ho reaches out to his contacts. This is a very important part of the show, because we learn in detail what Kang Dan-i was up against and why she had felt such despair.

> Cha Eun-ho meets with several recruiters who explain that a woman who left the workforce would simply not be considered

for a job. Her resume would be discarded because of the work break. Cha Eun-ho gets hysterical at the discrimination Kang Dan-i is facing, and he begins to fear her despair will return.

But the show is careful also to present what companies are up against—the violence of the free market, we might call it. We are frequently reminded of this anxiety when the president of Gyeoru, Kim Jae-min, asks his leadership team over and over, "Are we content to be number 5?" to which they, wagging their fingers, respond, "No, no, no."

We also see President Kim Jae-min talk about friends in the publishing industry whose businesses have failed. The costs of every error, the penalties for guessing wrong on how many books to print, the efforts to decode the design moves and marketing schemes that might help them get ahead—all of these are shown to us so that we have some idea of what is in the balance.

People speak about the *ppali ppali*— hurry, hurry—culture of Korea. I experienced this when I mused to my friend Eunju Hwang that I'd like a beautiful tee shirt like the one she was wearing, only redesigned to fit the Flexner lectures I'd be giving on my return from Korea. She said she'd organize the redesign and production of the tee shirts for me. I received a photograph the next day of the redesigned tee shirt and loved what I saw. Less than 48 hours later, the tee shirts arrived. We'd barely agreed on the design and they were done! *Ppali ppali* (Figure 4.2).

Ppali ppali shows up in *Romance Is a Bonus Book*: books appear speedily, like my tee shirts. South Korea didn't go from poor to wealthy simply as a gift from the US. The *people* did that by dint of extraordinary hard work. That hard work was pushed by the carrot of freedom from want and by the big stick of precarity.

Karl Marx made the capitalists spitting mad, probably because he explained that they don't get rich by working hard—they get rich by usurping the profits that come from the hard work of the rest of us. Capitalists still don't want us to know this secret, and can

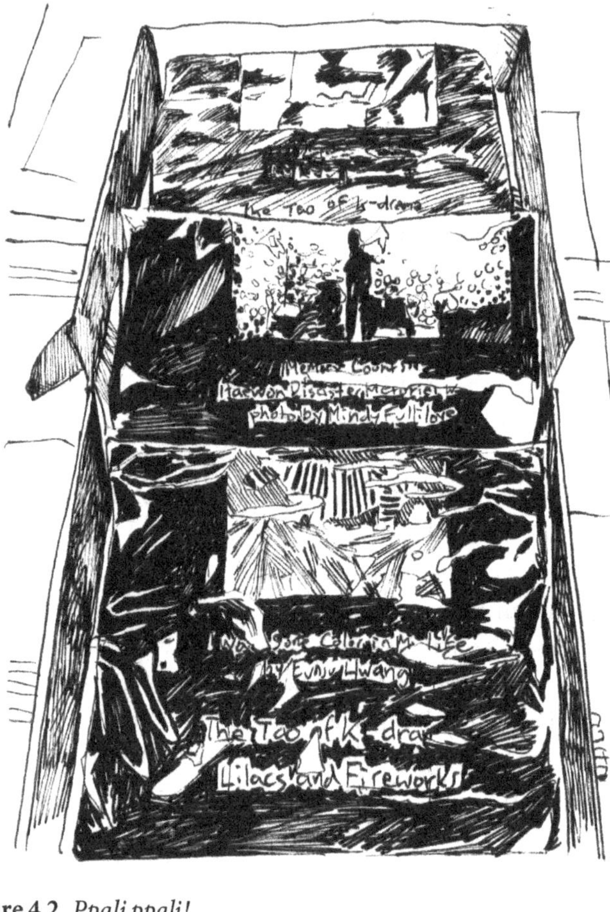

Figure 4.2 *Ppali ppali!.*
The three tee shirts that came quickly.
Drawing by Mike Malbrough, used with permission.

you blame them? If we really understood this process of "accumulation through dispossession," would we accept the grievous inequality that exists in the world today?

And yet, despite the ways in which we are exploited in the workplace—and maybe kicked and humiliated—we want to work.[5] Work makes us tired, but it also makes us feel a host of other things that are important. We work with others and we feel part of a team. We make something and we see it as a thing outside ourselves, something we helped to produce. We see this over and over in *Romance Is a Bonus Book*. The team at Gyeoru takes great delight in placing each new book on a platter and presenting it to the president, who picks it up, smells the fresh-off-the-press scent, and says, "I smell a best-seller."

When it's Kang Dan-i's turn to present the book, she joyously joins in the celebration and they laugh together. She is so proud to have been part of the process that led to the publication of a book. After she is forced out of Gyeoru, Kang Dan-i gets a job at another publishing company. This press is not honest or invested in their products. When she discovers that they plan to publish a plagiarized text, she points this out to the owner, who basically shrugs and says, "So?" Kang Dan-i knows what it is like to make a book ethically from her time at Gyeoru. To uphold those principles, she quits.

Work that is honest, creative, and sound imparts a host of good feelings. But I think even the worst kinds of work under the most terrible conditions can have meaning to people, and that meaning goes beyond the paycheck. We know that we did what was done. I am somebody because I can do this thing, horrible as it is; I can do it and I did do it.

There is an African American folk tale about a man named John Henry who worked on the railroad. He had terrific strength and could hammer the massive steel drill into the rock face faster than anyone. The company wanted to replace people with a steam drill. John Henry said, "Before I let the steam drill beat me down, I'll die with the hammer in my hand."[6] As the legend recounts, John Henry used two 10-pound hammers, one in each hand, to pound a 14-foot hole in the rock. The drill fell short by 5 feet. Thus, John Henry beat the steam drill; he later died of exhaustion.

This is a complex tale, rife with the struggles between workers and technology that define the struggle over labor rights to this day. It is a reminder of the contradiction between productivity and life. John Henry's pride in his work was something worth dying for. It is an exemplary moment showing the extreme sacrifices workers make to maintain their dignity. The tale is also a reminder that we must fight for life and dignity. If we don't, what will our lives be like?

Work is reflexive. I am presented with something to do, I do it, and when it is done I see—concretely and in real time—the difference I have made. It doesn't have to be that others see it or acknowledge it. Think of mathematicians who did work that sat for hundreds of years before others understood it. While the people who did the work might have appreciated acknowledgment from others, they knew, even if others did not, that they had solved the problem before them. They might even have felt a bit arrogant that they could do it and others couldn't. It's possible.

Work, I argue, is at the heart of our survival. We must find food to eat, water to drink, and people to love. We must raise our children, take care of our parents, and tend our homes. We must invent things. We must sing and dance and make fires. Work is like breathing. What may be a bit unnatural are relaxation and leisure—we are, by nature, busy bees.

And that is what Kang Dan-i wants in her life: she wants to work. She wants the team, the product, the challenge, and the paycheck. Her enthusiasm and talent change the Gyeoru company. She is a woman and a mother and she also wants to be a person who contributes in the workplace.

Cultural commentator Euny Hong has argued that K-dramas help us see why and how the heavy burdens on women are driving down the birthrate.[7] It was in large part from the show *Romance Is a Bonus Book* that I understood that romance is important to K-drama, but the resolution of the romance does not signal the happy end; it signals the shift to the work of the community to make the world better. In the terms of the Chinese philosophers, it's the time to put a better pattern on the world.

And the Winner Is . . .

Gyeoru held a contest, Tomorrow of Promise, for its employees to come up with new book ideas. Shortly after entering the contest, Kang Dan-i was pushed out of the company. She is gone when the day arrives on which they will announce the winner. Cha Eun-ho is operating the computer, so he sees the name first. He stands up and without saying anything leaves the room. He goes to the office kitchen and says, "*Oori* Dan-i," shaking his head with delight and doing a bit of the Powerdance. The others, back in the conference room, see what is happening and exclaim, "Oh. My. God."

President Kim Jae-min and other members of the leadership team realize the ways in which their system injured and abandoned this creative, delightful woman. They want her back. It is Associate Director Go Yu-seon—who gave her dry cleaning to Dan-i in the beginning—who points out the loophole. Drawing on the show's absurdist side, the president goes to find Kang Dan-i. The wind is blowing and his trenchcoat is billowing as he hands her his card and makes his recruitment speech. After a very short negotiation, they are giggling and high-fiving and Dan-i is *back*.

But that is not all.

The leadership changes its policies to welcome all kinds of people to the workplace. No one, they now understand, should have to suffer as Kang Dan-i did. Nor should they lose talent because of prejudice about who has it.

And that too is not all.

The company needs profit to survive; "I smell a best-seller" is not a joke. But the president affirms that publishing best-sellers permits them to publish "steady sellers," notable books that are not profit centers. This commitment had been in contention for the whole show, fears that are quieted by its affirmation at the party.

But wait! There's more!

> Kang Dan-i and Cha Eun-ho had kept their relationship a secret. But Cha Eun-ho takes her hand in front of the whole team, declaring that they are together. They run off as the song "Happy End" is playing.

But *wait*—the song that was playing as she went to her disastrous marriage? "Tell me now, *even lie*"?

The Door to My Heart

For me, one of the "secrets" of the show was hidden in plain sight: the two times the song is sung are two different versions! One is in English, sung by Lee Hae-min, and the other in Korean, sung by SAya and Kim Ki-won; both versions are written by Nam Hye-seung and her colleagues. The words do not represent a translation of the lyrics but two different sets of lyrics.

The English version plays as our heroine heads to her disastrous marriage in the opening of the show.[8] At the end of the show, as Eun-ho and Dan-i run off together, the song is sung as a duet in Korean. It was only when I had learned a little Korean that I realized the lyrics were not the same. The Korean version included the word "*oori*"—"we"—and I knew there was no "we" in the English version. I finally consulted the translation:

> One day you stood in front of the door to my heart . . .
> That's how our fairy tale started.[9]

I was so intrigued by this—and so convinced the two versions were also musically different—that I asked musicologist Dr. Margaux Simmons if she would analyze it for me. She emailed me:

The first time the song, "Happy End," appears it is sung by a female soprano voice in English. The text of this song expresses uncertainty and anxiety in terms like, "A little lost I am," and "Tell me now, even lie, it will be alright. Maybe things will turn out alright in the end." Her short solo is accompanied by piano alone and this exposition of the song is quite short.

When the song appears again at the end, it is sung as a duet, male and female singers. The key of the song has shifted to a half-step lower and the piano accompaniment has a lower, more prominent bass part. It also sounds as if the pedal is added to the piano, broadening and opening the texture from the beginning. The soprano begins singing solo in Korean but this time the text does not include words of uncertainty or questioning. The text begins with, "I guess it waited for a while, my heart, to recognize you. My heart has never beat like this before but now it's racing." A synthesizer joins the piano and the texture is further broadened and enlarged to include a higher musical range and adds an airiness that dramatically brightens the musical texture.

The male voice comes in singing solo, also in Korean, after the female voice has sung two verses. It's interesting that the first time the two sing together, they sing in English: "Oh when you say love. Here we go again." The male voice continues on alone in Korean for a few lines of text and then they both sing the remainder of the song together in Korean.

The synthesized sound added to the piano adds a light, spacious, ethereal quality to the whole song and imparts an uplifting mood. The ancient Greeks believed that certain tones imparted particular emotional qualities which they used in their ideology of "Music of the Spheres." Also, in Indian (India) musicology, there is the strong belief that certain ragas, or scales, impart definite moods and emotional states. I think Nam Hye-Seung may be tapping into this ancient wisdom for her song, "Happy End."[10]

Oori Jib (Our House)

The "door to my heart" is connected to the door of *oori jib*, our house. Kimchi Mamas, a group of women who are raising Korean and Korean American children, describe *oori* as follows:

> In Korean (and other Confucian-derived value system) culture, there is the concept of *oori*, which is a word that translates more or less into "us" or "ours." It permeates Korean societal order and dictates family roles and responsibilities. Often when one refers to her parents, she would say *oori um-ma, oori ap-pa*, "our mom," "our dad" instead of "my mom," "my dad," because no one singularly owns any relationship. *We all belong to one another.*[11]

Precarity fights against *oori*; *oori* fights against isolation. At one point in the show, Kang Dan-i uses "*oori*" to describe an activity she and the man she's flirting with did. Cha Eun-ho is furious. "You just met him—that's not *oori*. You and me, that's *oori*!"

My friend Sarah Howe taught English in Korea for five years and was there at the time of the 1997 financial crisis, called the "IMF crisis." The International Monetary Fund bailed the country out, creating a huge debt. Koreans were mortified by this collective debt. Sarah described watching people take their gold jewelry to banks to pay off the nation's debt.

During the hottest-up-until-then summer of 2024, the US government proposed that air conditioners be set to 78 degrees during the day and 82 at night. Responding to this news, Drew Garrison posted on Twitter, "Just know I'll let the entire power grid go down and ruin all of our lives before my thermostat is set at 78°."[12]

We have a long way to go.

5

Peace in the Neighborhood

Kim Je-hyeok Builds a Team

I needed to be in the belly of the beast, because now I can see that those who are closest to the pain need to have a seat at the table.

—Yusef Salaam, one of the Exonerated Five and NYC Councilman

"If we only have this day to live, let's live as human beings."

—Kim Min-cheol, *Prison Playbook*

In studying, there is a daily increase,
While in learning of way-making (*dao*), there is a daily decrease;
One loses and again loses
To the point that one does everything noncoercively (*wuwei*).
One does things noncoercively
And yet nothing goes undone.

—*The Tao*, No. 48

In the K-drama *Prison Playbook*, the acclaimed baseball player Kim Je-hyeok wakes up on a sunny morning in his apartment high above Seoul, a few days before he is scheduled to fly to Boston to join the legendary Red Sox. A breeze is ruffling the gauzy curtain to the left of the floor-to-ceiling windows that frame the view. He drinks a cappuccino, wipes the foam from his mouth, pulls a fine white dress shirt over his broad chest, and asks his doorman to hold the frozen abalone that has just arrived. "I'll be back soon," he says.

It's not that he doesn't know he's in a situation—that was announced when he saw a man attempting to rape his sister. Rather, it's that he's been assured that the consequence for beating the rapist will be probation and his life can go on as planned. So he puts on an elegant overcoat and heads to court. His lawyer is driving Kim's red sports car. By leaving through the underground parking garage, they are able to evade the press that is waiting at the front door.

But things do not go as planned. A voiceover tells us that Kim did not get probation as expected. Instead, he has been sentenced to a year in prison.

The Mazeway Breaks

What we see as Kim Je-hyeok arrives at the prison is that he is frozen in shock. He barely answers as a young man called "Jailbird" offers helpful information. In the intake room, Kim Je-hyeok sits without stirring while fights break out between rival gang members and officers rush in to control the situation. He barely murmurs as he endures the ignominy of officers rushing in to peek at his anal exam.

Impassive, he takes a green tub that contains his prison outfit, a toothbrush and toothpaste, and white rubber shoes. Dressed in the prison uniform and wearing the white shoes, he carries the tub down the hall of the cell block. Prisoners come to their windows to see him pass, whispering supportive comments.

These scenes of Kim Je-hyeok's struggle in the face of losing his way of life reminded me of a story told by anthropologist Anthony F. C. Wallace:

> One winter's day in 1649, a band of warriors from the Petun Indian village of St. Jean, south of the Georgian Bay, went out to intercept an invading war-party of Iroquois. They did not find the enemy. When they returned to the village, four days later, they saw only the ashes of their home and the charred and mutilated bodies of many of their wives, children, and old men. Not one living soul had escaped death or capture; not one cabin had been spared from the flames. The Petun warriors sat down in the snow, mute and motionless, and no one spoke or moved for half a day; no one even stirred to pursue the Iroquois in order to save the captives or gain revenge.[1]

The temporary paralysis, or shock, that Wallace described here is surprising because we expect that men of action will continue to be men of action. But confronted by this disaster, they cannot move at all. How and why can that be? Wallace reflected:

> Let us begin with a couple of analogies. They are liable to various qualifications, some of which I shall state, and which will be apparent both to psychologists and culturologists. One analogy is between non-material culture and "the way" a laboratory animal learns to run a maze in order to satisfy a want, like hunger. The other analogy is between material culture, natural environment, and persons and the maze itself. Human beings can be described as organisms whose peculiarity it is to construct and modify, slowly and laboriously, over centuries, very complicated sets of mazes for themselves and their posterity, with elaborate interconnecting doors and pathways; and also to construct complex rules for interaction and even mutual aid in operating the maze, as "the way" to satisfy their multifarious wants.[2]

The way of operating the maze—especially the particular way one person moves through the maze to satisfy wants—becomes the "mazeway," an object of our attachment. Wallace elaborated:

> Man, in other words, falls in love with his maze and his way of running it because they are associated with every satisfaction he derives from life, and, indeed, with the maintenance of life itself. The maze-way is "loved" whereas the "rewards" are merely enjoyed.[3]

The mazeway is both utilitarian, letting us move efficiently and effectively in the world, and beloved. It is a part of our understanding of ourselves. Students of the psychology of place would speak of these emotional connections as place attachment, sense of place, and place identification. The key is that the mazeway is embodied by the individual, guiding their every movement. The loss of the mazeway means the loss of the "how" to move. Even when the mazeway is lost as a result of an attack, the need to counterattack must take second place to the disorientation and grief that accompany the mazeway's loss. It is not obvious how to counterattack without the structuring elements of the mazeway. Wallace wrote:

> The identification of the individual with his culture can be disrupted under various conditions. One condition of disruption is sudden physical destruction of the maze itself, or of a part of it. In [that] case, the individual experiences a shock comparable to sudden and drastic bereavement, which temporarily interferes with his capacity to act with insight or to carry out such elements of his way as the remaining portions of the maze permit. His reactive depression is apparently disproportionate to the "real" situation: in other words, in a maze large enough for most visible (from a given point) portions to be destroyed or damaged without the whole maze actually being destroyed the destruction

> of part results in a reaction as if the whole maze were gone. The impact, furthermore, precipitates a regression to a very early, infantile, and primitive way, and the restitution of more mature learned ways should come about as he discovers, to his great joy, that the maze has not in fact been entirely destroyed after all.[4]

Wallace is offering a series of complex insights, each of which helps us decode the opening moments of *Prison Playbook*. There is no question that Kim Je-hyeok has experienced "a shock comparable to sudden and drastic bereavement, which temporarily interferes with his capacity to act with insight or to carry out such elements of his way as the remaining portions of the maze permit." Although his appeal will be heard in a week, Kim experiences that as an infinitely long period of time, during which he is given terrible food, forced to sleep in a room with five bizarre and dangerous men, and left vulnerable to extortion by corrupt authorities.

He counteracts his powerlessness by taking actions, perhaps to his own detriment.

> He is ushered into a cell with an array of men, including the strange "professor," a subservient old man, a ditzy young addict, a fat gangster, and the gangster's henchman Crony. When Seagull parades his domination of the subservient old man, Kim Je-hyeok's protective instincts are aroused but the other cellmates stop him before he can act, explaining that what Seagull is doing is OK in the ways of the prison.
>
> Kim Je-hyeok sits with this knowledge, but unable to tolerate it, he demands that the gangster get up and fight him. This assault threatens Kim Je-hyeok's chances of getting out on appeal. The warden offers to protect him for 30,000,000 Korean won (about $30,000). Kim has learned, however, that Jailbird, the young man who gave him helpful advice when he arrived, needs money for his mother's surgery. Kim sends money for her instead of to the warden.

Had he taken the long view, he might have accepted the abuse of the old man or given the warden the money. We learn that he has, in the words of his best friend Lee Joon-ho, "money to burn." But he is not able to accept those choices. Partly because of his character and partly because of shock—he has no long view—he cannot connect to his "mature learned ways" in these early days of his trials. And acting, however impulsively, assuages his feelings of destitution. It is an "I can" as a rebuttal to "No you can't."

Kim Je-hyeok has to learn that the whole of his mazeway has not been destroyed. He is famous, wealthy, and well loved by many, in particular by his ex-girlfriend, Kim Ji-ho, who is a student of Oriental Medicine; his best friend, Lee Joon-ho, a prison guard who is by his side throughout this ordeal; and Lee Joon-ho's younger brother, Lee Joon-dol, a sportswriter who will keep him connected to the outside world. The existence and assets of the larger mazeway are not obvious at the moment of the bereavement. It takes a period of adjustment for the larger whole to come into view and an even longer period of time for Kim to understand how to use it from the vantage point of his new position.

One complicated feature of the mazeway is that it is both an individual creation and a work of collectives over generations. A baby or a stranger is brought into the way of the maze in a particular place at a particular point in time. That is what happens to Kim Je-hyeok as he is imprisoned. As the title *Prison Playbook* suggests, there are instructions for living in prison. And indeed, beginning with Jailbird, people are giving Kim advice on managing life in prison. One peculiar piece of advice he struggles to understand is that religious services are a good place in which to scream—Jailbird tells him this, Lee Jun-ho tells him this, and a Buddhist monk tells him this. At the outset, Kim says to himself, "I don't want to scream—it's so loud." But at the point at which he absolutely needs to scream, he knows where to go.

The Playbook of Korea

People often ask me why I went to South Korea. I could have quoted Wallace's beautiful statement about the complexity of the Way and my desire to be in the flow of that. Instead, I answer, "I just wanted to go to a coffee shop and watch people go by," which seems a less technical equivalent. Anthropologists know what I'm saying; others are somewhat puzzled. An article in *Travel and Leisure* captured the hype of visiting South Korea and Seoul in particular, calling it the most beautiful city in the world, with fabulous palaces, outrageous dining, and fashion like nowhere else.[5] But that touristy stuff wasn't my interest: I wanted to feel the mazeway (Figure 5.1).

Mazeways have playbooks, and anthropologists are always looking for key informants to explain these playbooks. I too was looking for that and found that lots of people had advice. Eunju Hwang, a professor of English at Sogang University, gave me a series of books to read. When I commented on how dark they were, she explained, "I'm trying to show you the unconscious of Korea."

Dr. Lee Bora had the same message and took us to two revelatory places. The first was Seodaemun Prison, where anti-Japanese activists had been incarcerated, many of whom were tortured and killed.[6] The second was the War and Women's Human Rights Museum, which showcased the experiences of Korean women forced into sexual slavery by the Japanese Army.[7]

When I was having trouble with my arthritis, Dr. Lee referred me to Kim Ji-yong, a doctor of Oriental Medicine. The treatment, which got me back on my feet in record time, included advice on mazeways. "Have you seen the cherry blossoms yet?" Dr. Kim asked. I hadn't and was longing to. He offered, "Seoul National University is near here. There you can see a wonderful display of cherry blossoms."

He gave me careful instructions about how to get there. My goddaughter Gahlia was with me that day, so we followed his advice

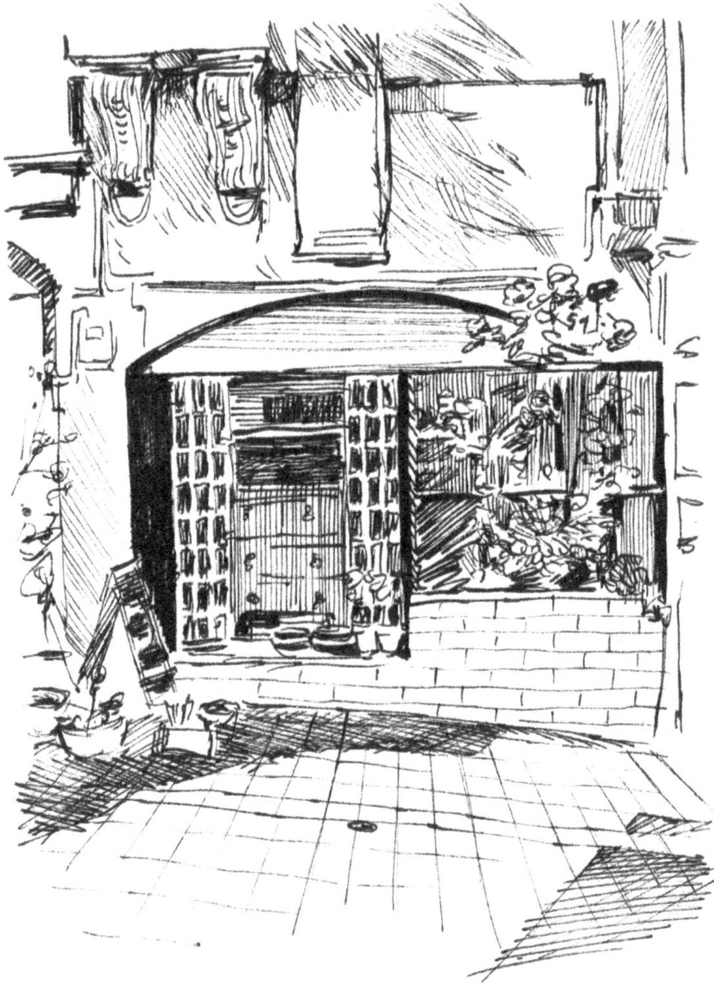

Figure 5.1 Min's Flower Shop.
A rose bush with lilac flowers grew from the window.
Drawing by Mike Malbrough, used with permission.

and quickly arrived at the famous Seoul National University, which was flanked by a park named in honor of Gam Gang-chan, a first-century military hero. In addition to the flowering cherry trees, we got to visit a site that honored him and told of his accomplishments. I am not a fan of selfies, but having learned about his courage and cleverness, I really wanted a picture beside the cartoon version of Gam Gang-chan, which Gahlia graciously snapped for me (Figure 5.2).

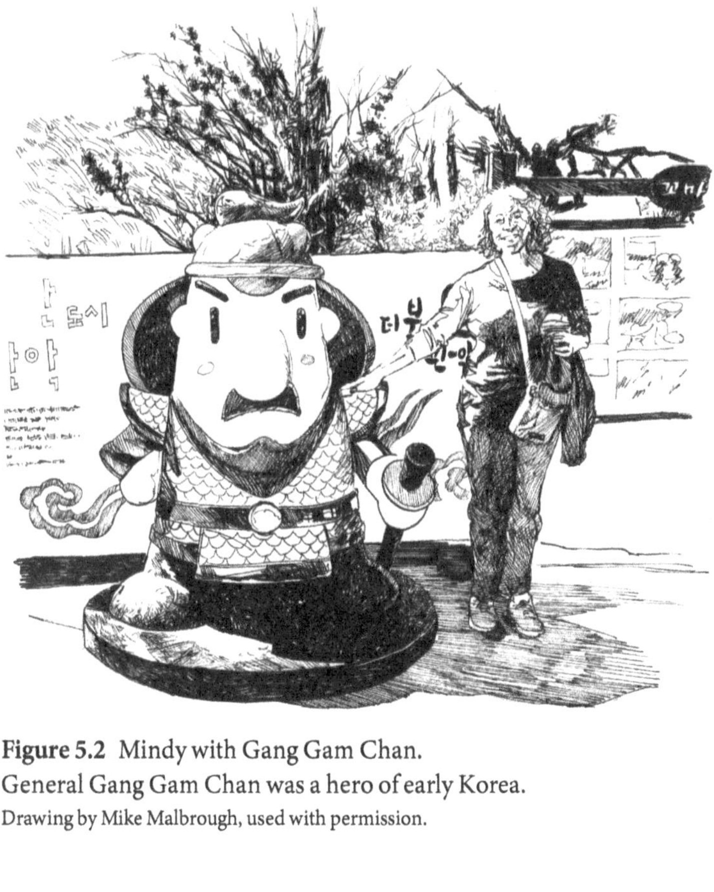

Figure 5.2 Mindy with Gang Gam Chan.
General Gang Gam Chan was a hero of early Korea.
Drawing by Mike Malbrough, used with permission.

Dr. Kim also advised Gahlia and me on places to eat, books to read, and exercises to do. His holistic approach to our care helped us to be healthy, which is deeply important in Korea, and to experience life from many points of view.

Kim Je-hyeok and the Prison

In the beginning of Episode 3, we find Kim Je-hyeok at Seobu Penitentiary, having lost his appeal. As in the US, where there are differences between jails and prisons, in Korea there are differences between detention centers and penitentiaries. The detention center is temporary, as people await trial. The penitentiary is the place in which one serves one's sentence—in Kim Je-hyeok's case, one year, and in other cases, for life. A doctor tells Kim Je-hyeok that it's different at the penitentiary: it's a rougher crowd, both prisoners and guards, and life unfolds on a different timescale.

A former prison, Jangheung, is used as the setting for *Prison Playbook* and other prison shows.[8] It is old and has many traces of the lives that were lived there. Scenes of the show—and this aerial photo—make clear that the prison is composed of many buildings, and the prisoners move among them. The cells in which groups of prisoners spend much of their time act as "homes." The prisoners regularly leave "home" to go to their work details, the infirmary, the auditorium, and the yard, among others. In those settings, we see interactions among prisoners from different cells. This movement within the neighborhood is essential to understanding the issue of making peace in the neighborhood (Figure 5.3).

In Korean the show title reads as "Wise Prison Life." The Wisdom that we will see is Kim Je-hyeok's movement from terrified newcomer, tub in hand, to what one witty recapper called a "prison gang leader." In this transformation, he shows his ability to learn the rules, create a group, and move the group in ways that help them live wisely under the duress of prison.

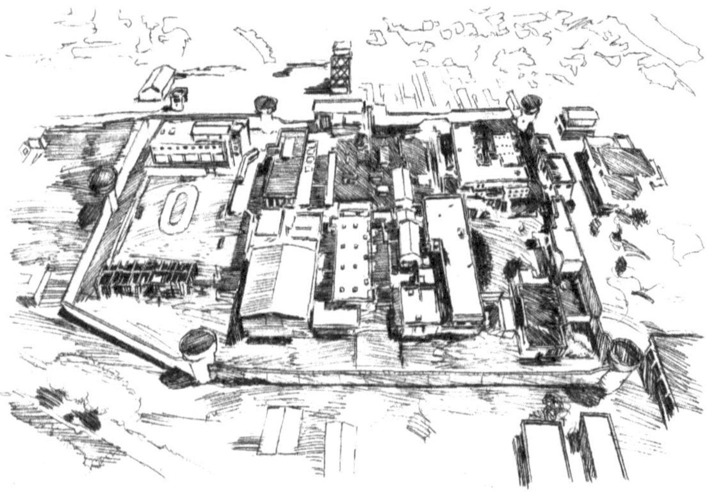

Figure 5.3 Jangheung Prison, Aerial View.
Jangheung Prison has been decommissioned and is used in movies and television shows that need its authenticity.
Drawing by Mike Malbrough, used with permission.

At Seobu Prison, Kim Je-hyeok is once again in a cell with other men. This group has been together for a while and has stable routines and even dreams. There is a long sequence in Episode 3 in which they whisper together. Kim Je-hyeok is not included in these conversations. A young man, nicknamed Jean ValJean because he stole bread, asks his mentor Minchul if he thought Kim Je-hyeok heard what they were saying. Minchul replies, "No, he wasn't listening."

The conspiring goes on all day and involves the errand boy and an unknown person, called Yong-shik. Minchul says to them all, "If we have only this day to live, let's live as human beings." Determined, he takes a hammer out of his Bible and gives it to the errand boy. "Kill Yong-shik if you have to."

We see the errand boy's silhouette banging away. And then the errand boy returns with a bag full of ramen, cooked, as it should

> be, in hot water, an item that is impossible to get in the prison. Yong-shik, it turns out, is the name of the engineer who designed the water heater. The errand boy needed to smash the protective plate bearing his name in order to raise the temperature on the machine.
>
> And now we get back to Kim Je-hyeok. The men gather around the table, deliriously happily with their noodles. One says, "What about him?" pointing to Kim Je-hyeok, who seems to be sleeping.
>
> They call him to join them. He throws off his blanket and we see that he is holding his chopsticks. He pulls them apart and dives in.

Slowly, it dawns on me, and perhaps other viewers, that Kim Je-hyeok always knows "what time it is," so to speak. In the first four episodes we see Kim Je-hyeok (1) protect an errand boy and take out a gangster, (2) help save Jailbird's mother, (3) be aware of "RamenGate," and (4) bring down the warden who tries to extort him.

The Outside Game

These moves will have costs and benefits, which is part of the playbook.

> The gangster he took down will have his henchman, Crony, attack him. Crony stabs him in his left shoulder, his pitching arm, with a sharpened toothbrush. Eventually the wound leaves him paralyzed. Overhearing the doctor say that the chances of recovery are almost zero, Kim Je-hyeok decides to announce his retirement.
>
> Lee Joon-dol, Lee Joon-ho's brother, the investigative journalist, is Kim's most devoted fan. He is devastated by Kim's retirement and decides to start a petition to urge Kim Je-hyeok not

to retire, with a goal of 10 million signatures. Lee Joon-ho says, "That's impossible!"

Lee Joon-dol replies, "Why? I already have a million."

It's unclear if Kim Je-hyeok knows about the petition, because his face remains neutral so much of the time. But people in the prison, including guards and prisoners, keep coming up to him and saying, "I signed the petition. You have to play baseball again."

This agitation from fans keeps Kim Ji-ho, Kim Je-hyeok's ex-girlfriend, and Lee Joon-ho questioning the doctors and keeps the doctors attentive to what Kim is saying and doing and what he's NOT saying and doing. Kim Je-hyeok is NOT opting for surgery that would give him immediate relief and permit him to live a normal life but would preclude a return to baseball. The chief surgeon is sensitive to this inconsistency—I'm retired BUT I don't want surgery—and interprets correctly that he hopes to play again. Kim Ji-ho, who is studying Oriental Medicine, the field of my doctor, Kim Ji-yong, discerns that the doctor has a plan to achieve this.

She also realizes that Kim needs a face-saving way to undo his retirement if he is to return to baseball: she proposes that his old coach, her deceased father, will come to him in a dream and say it is his wish, and she asks the guys in the cell to carry out this plan. They give Kim a sleeping pill. Then they stage-whisper to one another as they are setting up the "dream." The next morning Kim Je-hyeok announces that his coach told him in a dream that he was to return to baseball.

A few days later the guys discover the sleeping pills in the garbage. Ahh, Kim Je-hyeock!

Can't Win for Trying

There is much more pain ahead for Kim Je-hyeok, but in what is perhaps his darkest hour, on his birthday, he learns simultaneously that the man he assaulted has died, making him a murderer, and that the warden has arranged a place for him to train.

> Guards and prisoners are clapping for him, but he is coming apart. He suddenly starts to spew his pain: "Has anyone been unluckier than I have been? I had to come back from a career-ending car accident that killed my coach, and at the same time learned I had cancer and had to have 12 rounds of chemotherapy. I wanted to quit a hundred times a day, but I kept going. For three years no team would have me. Then I got on a team and thought maybe I could be happy. Now I'm a murderer—why? Why? *Why* has this happened to me?"
>
> He stalks off.

왜—why—is pronounced "way" in Korean and can be drawn out to give it emphasis. Men will drop their voices to give it bass notes of rage. It is a remarkable sound, and the translation into "why" lacks the sonic impact of a rage-filled "WAAAYYY?". It is this emotion suddenly spilling out of this stoic man that is shocking to one and all.

My friend, the poet Michael Lally, told me that at one period in his life he was depressed and angry as his acting career had come up short and he barely had money to raise his children. At one point he screamed at friends who were whining about much smaller problems. This outburst, however, cleared the air, the way a sudden thunderstorm can drop the temperature and the humidity on a hot summer day.

That was the effect of Kim Je-hyeok's outburst—he was ready to get back to baseball and to connect to the mazeway of the prison in a deeper way. He even shared his fears with his best friend, Lee Joon-ho, who listened attentively, said kind things, and then asked, "What kind of ego trip are you on? Just try."

That made Kim Je-hyeok laugh and feel like himself again: Kim Je-hyeok is inside the prison, but the Korean boy culture is not strikingly different, and so Joon-ho's mock attack was reassuring.

The shock of losing his mazeway and being thrown into another has upended Kim Je-hyeok at every level of his being. By screaming "Why?," he was able to share that with the group. He let them in, which is a way of asking for help, and from that no-longer-alone place, he could begin to get his bearings again, to see that the mazeway was not entirely broken, that Lee Joon-ho was by his side and would make silly boy jokes as needed.

In Korean storytelling, it is moments like these that really astonish me. They indicate that there is not a continuous cycle but a herky-jerky one, like a car with a flat tire going ker-blunk, ker-blunk, ker-blunk that has to come to a stop and get the tire inflated. That pause for intervention from powers greater than the self—and there are many—God and gods, of course, but also weather and tides, economies, gangs of friends, a single friend, love in all its guises, a moment of awe. This is the micro-kindness that the Chinese philosophers held up for us to see and understand.

One of the most remarkable manifestations of the work of kindness is the transformation of Crony.

> We first meet Crony at the detention center. He shows up at the prison and stabs Kim with a sharpened toothbrush—this leads to Kim Je-hyeok's loss of the use of his arm. Crony returns and the cellmates unite to protect Kim Je-hyeok, at risk of another attack. Suddenly Kim Je-hyeok—the man of action—can't take it anymore. He strides up to Crony and asks, "Are you an athlete?"
>
> Crony replies that he is.
>
> Kim Je-hyeok says, "Good. You can catch for me. Let's play."
>
> Crony, who has nerves of steel, is able to do something none of the other prisoners can: catch major league pitching. He becomes devoted to Kim Je-hyeok, and when Kim Je-hyeok is discharged, he says to him, "You were the first to treat me like a person."

Mazeway and Collective Consciousness

People living in a certain place know things about living in that place. That is the point of elaborating mazeways over generations. While the concept of the mazeway helps us understand the individual's internalized awareness of place, it also helps us understand the ways in which mazeways are shared and reflect collective aspects of consciousness.

My colleague Rodrick Wallace has pioneered work on collective consciousness that is a major extension of the field of social psychiatry.[9] Social psychiatrists are concerned with the effects of society on mental health. This has largely been conceptualized as effects on individual mental health. Wallace's work opens a new intermediate dimension of thinking, that of the ways in which our thinking is shared. The structure of society, he contends, acts to partition the thinking of groups. This has major effects on societal action and problem-solving.

We see this repeatedly in *Prison Playbook,* and it is devastating to watch. While we are constantly shown signs that say "Empathic reform," the Powers-That-Be in the prison have their own agendas and separate their decision-making from the prisoners' decision-making. The most dreadful incident to me—speaking as a physician—was the delay in treatment after Crony's attack had left Kim Je-hyeok with a paralyzed arm.

> The warden wants him to give an interview to the press saying that the prison is doing right by him. He refuses. Captain Na, who embodies the most vindictive ideas for managing a prison, tells the warden to deny him access to care until he agrees to the interview.
>
> Kim Je-hyeok, being a man of action and not willing to give in at such a moment, convinces Chief Yeom—a prisoner who is trying to coerce Kim to have sex with him—to hit him in the head

with a nail. Kim Je-hyeok is immediately sent to the hospital, and it turns out that nothing vital has been hurt.

Thank God—I get sick just thinking about what might have happened.

The point here is that the profound division between what the prison's Powers-That-Be think and what the prisoners think creates a desperate gulf. Kim Je-hyeok's telling another inmate to "hit me" is not an isolated case of a prisoner going on a rampage or using underhanded means to solve a problem. Nor is such thinking limited to prisoners: in all situations of marginalization and oppression, we see the Powers-That-Be using means to promote their own ends and the people who are under their thumb using whatever means they can to survive. An old saying among Black people is "The white man does as he pleases; the Black man does as he can."

It is obviously problematic if the prison authorities are going to play games with people's health. But there are other issues at stake as well. The prison is ultimately one place. By creating deep divisions inside it, the authorities have severed the prison's ability to act as a single place. It will, instead, function as many subparts. Should a situation arise—a typhoon or a fire—that requires unified action, it would be delayed or made impossible by those divisions. There are an infinite number of instances of this. Certainly, in my work documenting civic responses to pandemics, I've seen such divisions delay intervention, causing thousands, or tens of thousands, of unnecessary deaths.[10]

Prison Playbook teaches us deep lessons about the flaws in society that put us all at risk. In the epigraph to this chapter I quoted Yusef Salaam, who was wrongly convicted of rape. He was exonerated and elected to the New York City Council. At his swearing in he said, "I needed to be in the belly of the beast, because now I can see that those who are closest to the pain need to have a seat at the table."[11] And the need for that seat is to serve all of us, to complete the circle of representation, to give us the best possible hope for the future.

The Balm in Gilead

An African American spiritual has the words "There is a balm in Gilead to heal a sin-sick soul." The balm in Seobu Penitentiary is friendship. At the heart of the story is Lee Joon-ho's love of Kim Jeong-hyeok. Throughout the whole story, Lee Joon-ho stands by his friend, helping him get through. In turn, Kim Je-hyeok wins many people over to his cause, not because he is a great baseball player, but because he cares for people and helps them out. There are many scenes featuring Kim Je-hyeok helping someone through a dark hour. These people, in turn, help him. The flow of friendship tempers the deprivations and fears of prison life.

Friendship is the web that holds Kim Je-hyeok as he pays for his crime. It also enables him to become more open and perhaps less vulnerable to the kind of rage that led to the crime. A neighborhood is not the same as a circle of friends. The prison's rules, structure, and concentration of bad guys make it a very particular kind of neighborhood. But "Wise Prison Life" suggests to us that people can learn and grow even in such a neighborhood. For all of us outside of prison yet prison adjacent, we need to ask ourselves what that can mean for us.

I saw *Calls from Home*, a lovely documentary by Sylvia Ryerson about a radio station that was near a federal prison.[12] Communication between prisoners and their families was difficult because of the prohibitively high price of phone calls. Workers at the radio station realized they could help with this. On Monday nights, the station would broadcast calls from people who had loved ones in the prison. Although it was a one-way conversation, the expressions of love and hope meant the world to the people inside. In carrying out this work of connection, the radio station was teaching all of us about the meaning of "neighbor." This reminds me of the important reflection by Rabbi Joachim Prinz at the 1963 March on Washington:

> In the realm of the spirit, our fathers taught us thousands of years ago that when God created man, he created him as everybody's neighbor. Neighbor is not a geographic term. It is a moral concept. It means our collective responsibility for the preservation of man's dignity and integrity.[13]

6

Peace in the City

Lee Gang-du Re-members a City

We cannot heal the deep wounds inflicted during the era of racial terrorism until we tell the truth about it.

—Bryan Stevenson, Founder, Equal Justice Institute

How do you move on after a senseless tragedy, one that shackles you to the trauma for life for a fault that wasn't of your own doing at all?

—VarietyRecaps

Hold tightly onto way-making in the present
To manage what is happening right now
And to understand where it began in the distant past.
This is what is called the drawstring of way-making.

—*The Tao*, No. 14

Lee Gang-du, the protagonist of *Just Between Lovers*, was trapped for seven days in a collapsed building.[1] He emerges profoundly traumatized. Knowing this, we are unnerved but not surprised to see him as an adult use illegal pain medicine or take a sledgehammer to a so-called memorial to the 48 people who died in the catastrophe. As noted in the recap:

> How do you move on after a senseless tragedy, one that shackles you to the trauma for life for a fault that wasn't of your own doing at all? There isn't one answer and everyone has

> their own method. Sometimes, some don't even move on while others are desperate to brush it all aside. Medical technology has improved leaps and bounds . . . but is there a way to repair broken souls?[2]

Lee Gang-du, by taking responsibility and rebuilding the memorial he destroyed, will help the broken city re-member—that is, bring its parts together into a new whole. The tragedy is pushed out of its long stasis by the decision to build a biotech center on the site of the building collapse. The digging forces many people to face their losses, and the turning of the earth will deepen understanding and reveal buried truths. We talk about "clearing the air" and its importance in relationships: here, "clearing the rubble" is fundamental to healing.

"그년 사랑하는 사이"

It was the Variety Recaps post for Episode 6 of the show that directed my attention to the title and especially the word "사이."[3] The recapper noted:

> **사이** (pronounced "Sa-Yi") is a funny word that refers to that thing between two things, be it a gap or a relationship. You can use it to describe a physical gap between two mountains (aka, a valley) or the invisible bond between two people. **사랑하는** (pronounced "sa-rang-ha-neun") is actually the word "love" conjugated into an adjective, and so in this case, describes what kind of **사이** the relationship or the gap is. If I translate it, it might come out to be something like, "of love."[4]

My colleague Dr. Paul Browde explained to me that the idea of the "space between" is very important in the work of his teacher, couples' therapist Hedy Schleifer, who has explained:

> Our relationships exist in the space between us. This is not just a metaphor; it is biological. The space between two people can be open and clear, or it can be chaotic and polluted. We don't need words to understand this; we just know it. If you walk into a room where people have been arguing, you can sense it, you can feel the energy coursing between them. When the space between two people is clear, there is an intimacy of connection in which they encounter one another in the present moment. Time seems to stand still. This is what Martin Buber, the Jewish philosopher, called the encounter of the souls.[5]

Dr. Browde's couples work uses Hedy Schleifer's technique of creating bridges so that people can cross the gap between them. *Just Between Lovers* is delving into exactly this territory. The recapper pointed out:

> At the end of each episode just before the previews, this phrase **그 사이** (pronounced "geu sa-yi") appears too and it literally means something like "that relationship" or "that gap" and then it expands into "**그냥 사랑하는 사이**", which with all the information you have now can be translated into "just a relationship of love" or "just a gap of love", which is amazing, because it's like a summary of the progression between two people's feelings(?), relationship(?).[6]

Professor Park suggested that we could translate the opening of the sequence as "the gap," which certainly describes the state of affairs at the opening of the show. Then the end of the sequence can be read as "just a loving relationship," emphasizing "just," perhaps in the sense of "such"—such a loving relationship!

Watching the flow of the title sequence suggests to me that the story is telling us that "Just because love comes into the space between," love and life can prosper. The collapse of the building was a terrific centripetal force. Because of the failure of resolution of the harm, many relationships are held at a painful, frozen distance. The stirring of the ground will occasion a reworking of those relationships. Because love comes into the frozen space, the distance in the relationships can be bridged and the intimacy restored. People who work with trauma often use the expression "re-membering"—reconnecting split-apart members—to describe this process (Figure 6.1).

Restoration of the Urban Ecosystem

The story takes us into the lives of an important set of characters, but the collapse of a mall disturbs the whole city, and the peace of

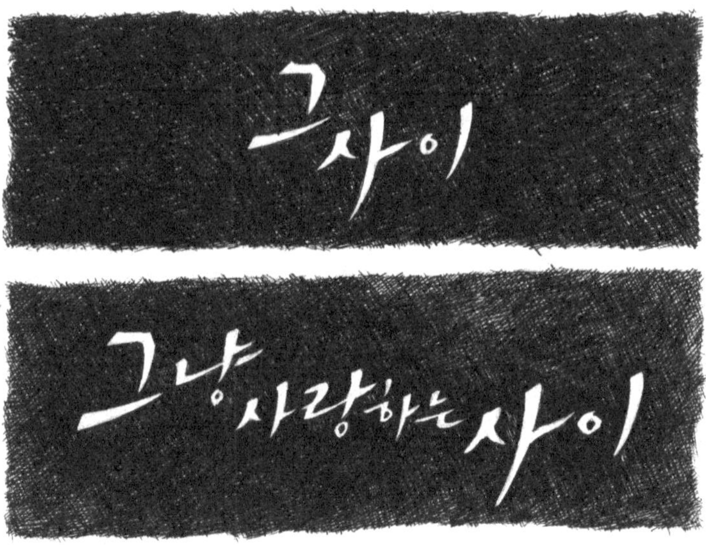

Figure 6.1 *Just Between Lovers* Opening Title Sequence.
The letters move apart and allow the word for love to change the phrase.
Drawing by Mike Malbrough, used with permission.

the city must be restored. Reverend Drew Jackson, in a homily on Jesus's message about peace, noted,

> When Jesus speaks of peace he has in mind the Hebrew concept of shalom. Shalom is not personal, inner peace, though that can be a byproduct of shalom. Shalom is a relational idea. It's social in nature. Shalom is when all parties in any given relationship are able to flourish and thrive in the fullness of who and what they were created to be.[7]

We cannot grasp the metaphor of rebuilding this single building without first understanding the rebuilding of the nation that had to occur after the Korean War. Bruce Cumings notes:

> Both Koreas were shattered by this fratricidal conflict, although the North suffered much more destruction in three years of intensive bombing than the South did in the nine months of warfare before the front stabilized in 1951. What the Japanese had begun with their massive shifts of Korean population in 1935–45, what the national division had intensified, the Korean War completed: Koreans of all classes were now thoroughly displaced from their local roots. Everyone was jostled or pushed or thrown bodily out of his or her social niche.[8]

With the help of other socialist countries, North Korea was rebuilt as a socialist state. North Korea's economy developed for the first couple decades after the war but then collapsed. Its evolution into the harsh militarism of the Kim dynasty was predicated on the vast destruction of the country during the war. With every village leveled, they clearly saw—and still see—American militarism as the enemy and prepared themselves should they have to face it again. Spending all one's money on the military has devastating costs for the rest of the economy, as the US has demonstrated.[9]

South Korea, under US influence, rapidly evolved as a capitalist nation. Without question, the South Korean people collectively rallied to rebuild their country and make it a world economic powerhouse. The "capitalist miracle" of South Korea is generally dated to 1961, when a coup d'état overthrew the vicious and corrupt Syngman Rhee and installed Park Chun Hee as president.[10] The authoritarian state established a partnership with the chaebol—the family conglomerates that came to dominate Korean industry—to direct and support the growth of industry, with an eye to international exports. Park's government—and the authoritarian regimes that followed—governed with both an iron fist and a velvet glove. They suppressed people's movements and labor unions but also realized they needed to co-opt enough public support to get people to work with fervor for the national project of development.[11] People routinely worked 12 to 16 hours a day, six days a week, usually for very low pay.

It is clear that the ethos of "work to be done"—할 일—dominated people's understanding of their life situation. The man who picked me up from the airport when I first landed in Incheon in February 2023 explained that they were afraid they would starve if they didn't all pitch in to set the country on its feet. He described the hours he worked and what it had cost his family. He never had time for his wife and children: on Sundays, his day off, he'd be so tired that he would just sleep all day. It was what everyone did, and he was obviously proud of his contribution. Gesturing to the high-rise apartments on either side of the highway, he noted that none of that existed before—he had been part of making it happen.

My driver's story alerted me that it was the sacrifices of the many that were making life better. At the same time, capitalist individualism fed off of old neo-Confucianism to promote the expectation that education was the key to the future. Competition for the scarce places in the "best schools" became part of national life—success in education meant hard work but decent pay, while not succeeding meant even harder work at low-paying part-time jobs, housing insecurity, and fear. While Seoul shines, the people within it are experiencing various kinds of trouble—including economic inequality, a high cost of living, a lack of decent job opportunities, and a lack of affordable housing. Precarity, as Kang Dan-i's story showed us, is real and pressing.

Among other kinds of fallout, we find the "big three": South Korea has the world's lowest birthrate,[12] a very high level of alcohol consumption,[13] and the highest rate of suicide among countries in the Organisation for Economic Development and Co-operation.[14] My driver shared that his children were well educated and successful but he doubted that he would ever have grandchildren.

The country has also experienced disasters, in which the chaebol cut corners to make even more profit or the government neglected warning signs and failed to protect the people. *Just Between Lovers* is taken from that story-fabric, which includes the 1995 collapse of a multistory department store that killed 502 people,[15] the Seowol ferry disaster in 2014 in which 304 people died,[16] and the Halloween disaster of 2022 when nearly 160 people were crushed to death.[17] These tragic events endure in the minds and bodies of the people of South Korea. Their ripple effects of grief and horror are part of the collective consciousness.

Because we need to see the scale of such an injury to truly understand it, the bus becomes a particularly important actor in the series. Buses, the primary mode of transit for many in Korean cities, are a crucial symbol of urban working-class life. They are how we move among the many characters and plots of *Just Between Lovers.*

Figure 6.2 shows the lead characters, Ha Mun-su and Lee Gangdu, at the center. They each enter with a set of relationships, which over time become interconnected. Because the problem involves so many people in their separate spaces, the scale and movement of this story are much greater than we saw in *Romance Is a Bonus Book,* which took us between home and office, or *Prison Playbook,* which took us around the neighborhood of the prison. *Just Between*

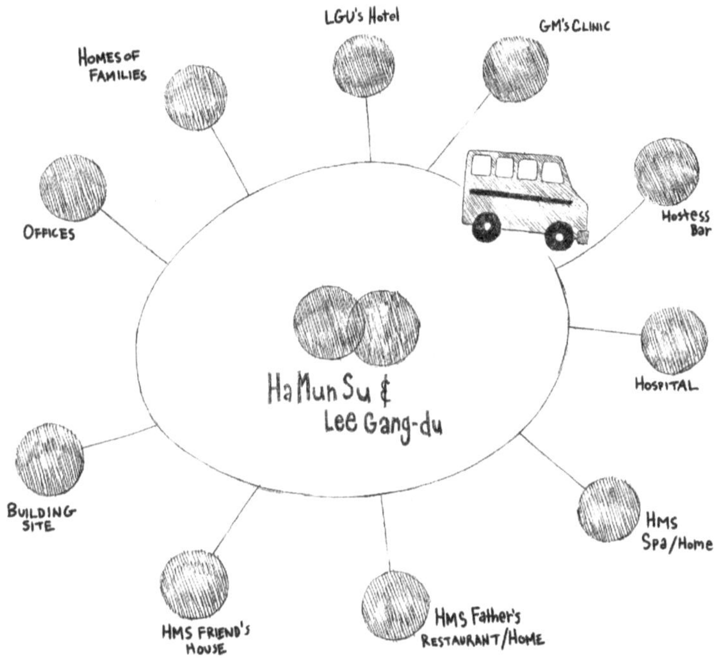

Figure 6.2 Lee Gang-du and Ha Mun-su Take the Bus.
The bus is central to life in Korean cities, and the movement of the bus anchors us in the scale of the intervention of the show.
Drawing by Mike Malbrough, used with permission.

Lovers takes us all around the city, mostly by bus. At each of the stops we see the relationships slowly come unstuck and the collective recovery launched by the rebuilding of the physical site and the development of the memorial. The psychic, social, and material excavation and rebuilding are what draw Lee Gang-du and Ha Mun-su together to re-member the city.

"Clearing the rubble" has a special meaning in Korea. People sit on the ground or on the floor all the time. In K-drama, when people are upset, they fall to the floor or the ground, even if there is a chair or a low wall nearby. We also constantly see people wiping the floor or sweeping the yard. The caretaking of the ground is of high importance. This relates to people changing their shoes as they enter a home or a school or even some offices. In *Misaeng*, when our hero Jang Geu-rae has to make a presentation, he uses the slippers of one of his coworkers as a prop. The slippers evoke body memory from everyone in his audience, their hearts open to him, and, against the odds, he wins the day.

Lee Gang-du and Ha Mun-su: The Effort to Be Free

The central characters in the show are Ha Mun-su and Lee Gang-du, two young people who were trapped together in the rubble of a collapsed building when they were 15, 10 years before the drama begins.

> Early on in the show, Lee Gang-du knows that Ha Mun-su is the girl he was trapped with in the rubble of the mall's collapse. She, however, has amnesia and doesn't remember him. He is shocked by this. Further, he has held a resentment against her for those 10 years, thinking that she escaped first and failed to tell anybody he was still there, leaving him trapped for four more days. Indeed, when he had insisted she be rescued first, because he knew she was dying, he urged her to be sure to let them know he was there. What he doesn't know is that, during her rescue, she attempted to signal that he was there but was too weak to make herself heard. Then she was dropped on her head and lost her memory.
>
> Two kinds of motion—of body and mind—begin the healing.
>
> Lee Gang-du, who fights all the time, gets in the face of a former boss whose thugs beat him up and leave him in an alley. Ha Mun-su happens to be passing at the time and sees the men exit the alley. Their carriage worries her and she enters the alley

> to see what had happened there. She finds Lee Gang-du and kneels down by his side. He grabs her arm and clings to it.
>
> Her rescue of him triggers his curiosity. He wants to know who she is—perhaps recognizing that he knows her from the rubble. Because of his attention to her over the next few days, he is aware when she is missing, having fallen into a pit at the building site. She is feeling like she will die there, when Lee Gang-du, who has been searching for her, arrives at the pit. He pulls her out and she falls on him in the process; they look deep into each other's eyes and then scramble apart—a major tell of future love in K-drama. She begins to follow him everywhere. He asks her if she wanted to die in the hole. She says no, but she was prepared to die because she thought she might. She thanks him for saving her and becomes devoted to him.

In that early period, Lee Gang-du experiences torment. He exhibits clear signs of posttraumatic stress disorder: he has vivid flashbacks of the collapse and his time in the rubble; he has nightmares; he has a hair-trigger temper; and he has constant pain from his physical problems. He hallucinates the voice of Sang-jae, a teenager who died next to him in the rubble. Because Lee Gang-du's father died in the crash, for which he was not compensated, and his mother died of cancer thereafter, he has assumed responsibility for his younger sister. He works temporary jobs, toughened by the streets but known to be kind and loyal, which has won him many friends. To manage the contradictions of his situation, he takes blue pills, painkillers that are toxic to the liver. He is warned repeatedly that he shouldn't take so many and that he should go to a doctor, but he doesn't heed these warnings.

Why does Lee Gang-du remain bound to his trauma, and how is it by clearing the ground that he and others heal? The work of the Reverend Dr. Grace Ji-Sun Kim, a theologian at Earlham School of Religion, was very helpful in answering this question. Her book enticed me because it had "*han*" in the title: *The Homebrewed*

Christianity Guide to the Holy Spirit: Hand-raisers, Han, and the Holy Ghost. Han is a perplexing word for me and other non-Koreans. Reverend Dr. Kim explains, "The Korean word *han* is difficult to translate into English. Two of the best translations are 'unjust suffering' and 'piercing of the heart.' *Han* is immense pain and suffering perpetrated by an individual, a group, or a situation. *Han* tries to express the painful tearing apart of one's heart due to injustices."[18]

Given this definition, it is fair to say that Lee Gang-du is suffering from *han*, both because he felt that Ha Mun-su had abandoned him in the rubble and because of his guilt at surviving when Sang-jae did not. He is paralyzed by these opposing feelings, unjust suffering on the one hand and shame on the other. He is trapped in a cycle of acting out his anger, medicating his pain, and regretting his actions. Reverend Dr. Kim goes on to propose that Spirit—whether we use its Christian name "Holy Ghost" or its Eastern name "Chi"—releases *han*.[19] In Oriental medicine, the stasis of Chi is recognized as a major cause of illness, and that is what we see in the case of Lee Gang-du. In my view, we learn first that root shock causes *han* and second that *han* is the reciprocal of restoration, the pain inversely related to the state of repair.

Gratitude and curiosity are two forms of the movement of Chi. Each breaks up hopelessness and resignation. It is not the case that in the early period of the show all is well with Lee Gang-du and Ha Mun-su; rather, a small crack has appeared in the posttrauma *han*. Healing begins. It has to have ups and downs, because that is how recovery works, in a zig-zag rather than a linear progression from hurt to wellness. But it is in the connection that has been made by the two rescues that love blossoms and the healing proceeds, in its own way, to a happy ending.

The movement of Spirit, in the Christian tradition, represents God's grace. In the dialectics of the *Tao Te Ching*, movement is the heart of the universe. The Tao advises against coercive action, trusting instead that the movement of the world is always creating change. We need to see and understand and move with the flow of that.

> As he connects to Ha Mun-su, Lee Gang-du begins to shift. He realizes that she didn't abandon him but rather suffered a traumatic brain injury, and he is able to let go of his resentment and love her instead. He starts to think about the next day, if not further into the future. He wants to see her and to be with her. He is delighted by her, and this awakens hope in him. And he is fascinated by the bits of the knowledge that peek through her amnesia. For example, she recites a complex soccer story that he'd recounted to her, even though she has no idea why she knows that, and only that, story about soccer.
>
> More and more of Ha Mun-su's memory returns as the show progresses. She remembers, first, that Lee Gang-du was there too and that they took care of each other. Later, when she has regained all her memories, she is overwhelmed by the idea that, by her failures, she contributed to Lee Gang-du's suffering and the deaths of Sang-jae and her little sister. She runs away from Lee Gang-du—being with him stirs up her angst. He affirms repeatedly that it was not her fault, filling the space between them with his love.

This is one of the major lessons about the way in which love enters the newly opened space and helps to solve problems, whether it is lifting guilt, facing the truth in a balanced manner, or taking on other tasks of healing trauma. We see, in this relationship, the way re-membering works in this story—bringing parts of the story back together and learning to have compassion for the messy whole.

Ha Dong-chul and Yoon-ok: Who Is to Blame?

In the aftermath of their older daughter's amnesia and their younger daughter's death, the parents, Ha Dong-chul and Yoon-ok, are both bereaved and furious, with nowhere to put their anger.

They separate and she becomes an alcoholic. Ha Mun-su tenderly puts her mother to bed and clears away the soju bottles.

Her father, Ha Dong-chul, runs a noodle shop near the site of the disaster. Lee Gang-du, in trying to find out who Ha Mun-su is, goes to the shop and quickly puts the pieces together. He understands the current of depression that characterizes the father, who hasn't let go of his rage and his despair.

Seo Joo-won and Jung Yoo-jin: "Lies, Damned Lies and Statistics"

Why did the building collapse? This is the major problem that the story must uncover to prevent a recurrence of disaster.

> Seo Joo-won's father was the architect of the earlier building and said that it was his mistake. But we learn through flashbacks and overheard conversations that he was asked to take the fall for the sake of the construction company and the many jobs it provided. After being attacked by Ha Mun-su's father Ha Dong-chul, Seo Joo-won's father committed suicide. At that time, Seo Joo-won loved Jung Yoo-jin, the daughter of the company's owner. Seo Joo-won overheard her ask his father to take the blame for the building collapse and thus she was the proximal cause of his death. He cannot love her after that.
>
> But what was the real reason for the building's collapse?
>
> Jung Yoo-jin says to Seo Joo-won, "You and I both know the plans were perfect." Thus, the issue was in the execution. Though during the new construction Seo Joo-won is fighting against the kinds of wrongs that led to the collapse, he wavers in his determination. It takes Jung Yoo-jin, Ha Mun-su, and Lee Gang-du to keep him on course. Eventually he provides Jung Yoo-jin with the details of what her brother had approved that could lead to new harms. She pushes her brother out and takes over the company.

She acknowledges the mistake that led to his father's death and accepts responsibility for the outcome of the new building. However, she will never win Seo Joo-won back.

From Rage to Remembrance: The Memorial

The first few times I watched *Just Between Lovers*, I missed the importance of memorial making. It is a project that brings Lee Gang-du and Ha Mun-su into deeper relationship, creates pressure for honest rebuilding, and offers healing for all involved. It is the heart of the show. It reminds me of Bryan Stevenson, who created the Lynching Memorial in the US, who said, "We cannot heal the deep wounds inflicted during the era of racial terrorism until we tell the truth about it."[20]

In the first episode, we see a stone carved with the names of the 48 people who died in the collapse, including Mun-su's sister Ha Myeong-Su, her first love Sang-jae, and Lee Gang-du's father. We see Lee Gang-du take a sledgehammer to the memorial and destroy it. This is a coercive action, one for which he makes amends by offering to make a new memorial. He asks that Ha Mun-su work with him. In the following episodes, we see them visit a stone mason to ask about stones and carving. We see them search out other memorials, one of which is lost in the woods and obviously never visited by anyone.

There is an important pivot triggered by Lee Gang-du's best friend Sang-man, who comments that people are compassionate and that is why they care about cats. This makes Lee Gang-du reflect on the memorial. He realizes he and Ha Mun-su are on the wrong path: they're supposed to be comforting the bereaved. They begin to visit family members of those who died to ask about their loved ones. They have a variety of experiences, and they—and we—learn how a disaster shapes lives a decade after the event.

> The visits culminate in one to the mother of Sang-jae, the youth who haunts both of them. Lee Gang-du sees a picture of Sang-jae as a teenager laughing with his friends and says to his mother, "I thought he was scary." The mother weeps. Ha Mun-su mumbles, "I'm sorry, I'm sorry, I'm sorry." The visit helps to lay the ghost to rest for all three of them. Later, when Ha Mun-su is reflecting on when she started to love Lee Gang-du, she thinks of his singing to her in the rubble. The place is no longer associated with her proposed meeting of her first love, Sang-jae. It is now all about Lee Gang-du.

Memorials as Social Statements

Lee Gang-du and Ha Mun-su reclaim a pillar from the landfill for the memorial, with the intention of adding words about each lost person. They also design the garden in which it will be placed. The process is crucial not only to the recovery of memories but also to the role of watchdog that they play in keeping the company and the architect honest. The memorial, by bringing the voices of the lost into the open, into a prominent place in the site, acts to prevent future harm. Ha Mun-su and Lee Gang-du work to make the preventable collapse of a building part of the ethical commitment of all involved in the site.

Lee Gang-du's granny leaves him a piece of land that is essential to the biotech site. This puts him in the position to demand a central place for the memorial. Because corruption lines the pockets of powerful people, there is a lot of opposition from the top. It takes the strong collaboration that has grown among the four young survivors to bring the whole vision to light, as both monument and driver of honest behavior. That teaches us something important about memorials—they represent the images and ideas that people agree should be in the public space.

The design of the memorial pillar, its prominent placement, and its garden setting also teach us something about the ways in which memorials work. Of the many memorials I have visited and studied, it is Maya Lin's Vietnam Veterans Memorial on the Mall in Washington, DC that is the outstanding example of what a memorial can do. I happened to be treating a Vietnam veteran at the time the memorial was opened to the public. My patient was frozen, unable to access his emotions. He went to the ceremony and cried with other veterans. Finally, he, like others, felt that his pain and sacrifice were seen by his nation. He thawed and was able to be present in his life in a new way. There are many features of Maya Lin's masterpiece that contribute to this experience, I believe. At the heart of her teaching is that the memorial has to bring all of us into its space: those who died, those who are bereaved, and those of us who were not directly bereaved but need to see what happened.

A visit to an extraordinary garden helped me to see this in the Korean context. Byun Jeong Dae-seob is an artist who works in a small village near Gwangju. He is preoccupied with expressing what Professor Eunju Hwang described as "the unconscious of Korea," the deep, deep hurts of its long history and complicated present. Dae-seob Sem—"sem" is the title given to one's mentors or teachers—invited Gahlia and me to visit as part of a trip we made to see his neighbors, Doctors Howard Waitzkin and Mira Lee.

Sem's garden is a small, walled space that is exquisitely and constantly curated with layers of meaning and beauty. Spring was more advanced in the south, and lilacs and lots of other flowers were blooming. He explained to us many of the images and artifacts that were nestled here and there, like the painting of his dog on the wall of the small building he used as his studio. At one point in the afternoon, he pulled out a set of paintings and showed us his work. One painting was a Buddha-like face with a yellow ribbon, the symbol of the Sewol ferry disaster, which had shaken the country and still smarted because it was so badly handled by the government. Sem, standing in his garden holding up the painting for us to see, perfectly exemplified what Maya Lin accomplished and what Lee Gang-du is attempting to accomplish: telling the truth of a disaster in a setting so perfect and so impossible to miss that we are both comforted and confronted, able to feel and process the grief, rage, and love that are represented there. The power of this experience was what led me to propose that painting for the cover of this book.

Convergence

The movement of the show will bring people into contact with one another in new ways, enabling the healing to unfold. This convergence is beautifully represented in a scene that focuses on Lee Gang-du's granny, a cantankerous older woman who serves as an elder to the orphaned teenager.

> Granny runs an illegal clinic for people who can't get care through the formal system. When she becomes ill and is hospitalized, many people gather. Lee Gang-du is there, of course, and so is the owner of the hostess bar and Sang-man, Lee Gang-du's dear friend from his hotel. Lee Gang-du's sister, a trainee at the hospital, is taking care of Granny. Ha Mun-su has also come to know Granny and is there. Han Mun-su's wheelchair-bound best friend comes, accompanied by the young man who helps her navigate the world. Granny offers soda and candy from her stash as the women get their nails done. Granny enjoys the moments with all these good people.
>
> After Granny's death, there is a spontaneous gathering at her clinic, which turns into a memorial repast. People share snacks and memories of Granny, sorting out "who she really was" through their conversation. People have come from many different parts of the city to the clinic, which is located in a narrow alley.

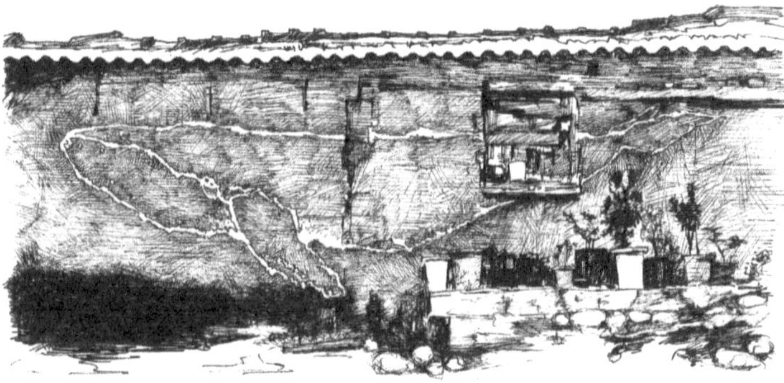

Figure 6.3 Dae-seob's Whale.
Byun Jeong Dae-seob painted this whale on the side of his house.
Drawing by Mike Malbrough, used with permission.

We see, as people connect and reconnect, how networks grow and change. And we see how the movement of Chi—of grace—permits people to move out of their frozen state and begin to live again.

Choosing Life

Lee Gang-du is slowly emerging from the trauma that shaped his life, but a crisis comes when his pill taking catches up with him and his liver fails. He needs a transplant in order to live. The doctors are shocked at how many people ask to be tested as a candidate to make an organ donation for him. None work out, and Lee Gang-du is very near death when a donor is found.

In the final scenes, we see that Lee Gang-du is studying for a test, which means he is planning for his future. He takes care when crossing a street because he knows Ha Mun-su would be sad if anything happened to him. We see people around the city getting invitations to the unveiling of the memorial; people whose stories we have come to know open their envelopes and smile, revealing both the breadth and depth of this city story.

The show ends at Ha Mun-su's home, which she is renovating, a handy metaphor for the show. With Ha Mun-su by his side, Lee Gang-du is able to say, "살아남아서 다행이다." The straight translation is "Thank God I survived." But, in light of all that has happened, I think a better translation is more idiographic. Drawing on the saying from Twelve Step Fellowship, "Don't leave before the miracle happens," I translate what Lee Gang-du is saying as "I am glad I waited for the miracle to happen."

We started this chapter with the recapper's question, "Is there a way to repair broken souls?"

The answer offered by this show is "Yes, there is. Chi opens the space so that love can come in and do the work it does so well."

7

Peace in the Nation

Dam-i Takes on Evil

> You must never be fearful about what you are doing when it is right.
>
> —Rosa Parks, US civil rights activist

> And upon taking the throne, the preceding king attempted to rule the nation with the highest form of benevolence in history for the better[ment] of the people.
>
> —Shin Young-soo, *The King's Affection*

> Know the clean
> Yet safeguard the soiled
> And be a valley to the world.
>
> —*The Tao*, No. 28

The King's Affection is an extended meditation on the moral arc of the universe and the obligations of good people to bend it toward justice.[1] Here's where my understanding of the show starts, with Chapter 53 from the *Tao Te Ching*:

> Their court is impeccably clean
> Yet the fields are overgrown with weeds
> And the granaries are empty . . .
> This is called highway robbery (*dao*)
> Which ought not to be confused with way-making (*dao*).[2]

The show poses exactly this scenario to Dam-i, a very principled young woman, and asks her to fight for way-making, not robbery. She is to carry out this task while disguised as a prince, hiding her identity and gender from her true love, fighting her evil grandfather, calling righteous people to help her, losing all but not giving up—I could go on. We are reminded of the old joke about Fred Astaire and his dancing partner Ginger Rogers: she did everything he did but backwards and in heels.

At every step Dam-i must make a moral decision, and her courageous decisions teach us the process of getting back to the Tao, the Path of a righteous life. Crucially, although burdened with the power and responsibilities of her role, she is not alone in her journey. Deep and challenging friendships mark the main road and accompany her on her moral path.

The show opens with the birth of twins, which, contrary to what we believe today, was thought to be an ominous sign. The fact that the boy had shared the womb with a girl was especially disastrous for his standing as king of Joseon, a highly unstable position to hold in the best of circumstances. The children's grandfather, who is mad for power, orders the murder of the girl. Their mother, with the help of her allies, sends the girl away from Hanyang, what we now call Seoul, so that she can live.

Dam-i, as the girl is known, grows up in a monastery until the monk who raised her dies. She then makes her way to the capital, where she lives in a slum with other orphans and begs on the street to survive. Her bright smile attracts a woman passing by, who takes her to the palace to be a court maid. Eventually Dam-i encounters her brother, Prince Lee Hwi, who looks just like her. On a particularly desperate day, he changes places with her. The resemblance has become apparent to the grandfather's minions, and they set out to kill Dam-i. Not realizing that the child dressed in maid's clothing is the prince, they murder him. Dam-i, meanwhile, is dressed as the prince. Her mother insists that she continue the masquerade to prevent many more deaths. Thus ensues a charade that will go on for 10 years. The story picks up at that point.

Three Moral Youths

This could be a story of ends-justify-the-means political machinations—one faction against another. But it is not. It is a story that pits respect-for-all-life against everything-is-mine, Dam-i's morality versus her grandfather's greed and ambition. An incident early in the show clarifies Dam-i's morality. She kneels to help a maid who broke a bowl. Her mother, the queen, scolds her and tells her not to help, care for, or get close to others. Dam-i responds, "But I don't want to live like that." And then we see the predicament Dam-i is in: the Queen responds, "It's the only way you'll survive." Faced with these terms, the young Dam-i shivers and retreats into herself, not conceding the point but hiding what she values from superior authority.

Over the course of the show, we learn only a little about the source of her values. We know that she was raised on a mountain by a monk and was used to being alone. We learn that she had great pity for the orphans who lived in the slums. We also learn that her bright smile and optimism, in spite of her hard life, won the heart of Jung Ji-un, her childhood sweetheart, and that her empathy for the poor touched him so deeply that he dedicated himself to their cause and hers.

In addition, we see that Dam-i enters into her masquerade knowing how to read a large number of Chinese characters. She has to read on her first encounter with the King. This is a critical part of her survival, because the prince was tutored by many people, and sudden illiteracy would have been an insurmountable challenge. It takes a lot of time to learn enough Chinese characters to be able to read the key Confucian texts the prince was studying, so mastering Chinese characters must have been part of her life at the monastery—though not the Confucian texts themselves: in one encounter with her father he asks her about one of the texts, and she is unable to answer. She had most likely read Buddhist texts at the monastery, and we can surmise that they are the source of her firm moral grounding, concern for others, deep respect for life, and commitment not to harm other beings.

I think we can also assume from her bright demeanor that she was loved and protected. Though the transition to her new life is a huge leap, she does not enter it as a traumatized child with rigid defenses, unable to adapt. She takes to the task and perseveres. It is a paradox that this very moral child is asked to live a lie. She has no choice in the matter at the start but quickly discerns a compromise: to live the part for a while, to abdicate in favor of her stepbrother as soon as she can, and to accept whatever punishment is given to her as a result of the deceit. She never suggests that she should be forgiven because she was thrust into the role.

She is what Victorian texts called "high-couraged."

Into this clash of values come two young men, both of whom have loved Dam-i since she was a child. One is Jung Ji-un, her childhood sweetheart. During their brief childhood romance, she saved his life because she knew how to swim and he did not, and she chastised him for not knowing the fighting arts. This, and her concern for the poor, shaped his life. He in turn gave her a name, Yeon-seon, which he thought a better fit than Dam-i.[3]

Jung Ji-un is deeply hurt by the twins' tragedy. He loses Dam-i, who is hidden by her transition, and he also sees his father kill a young girl to cover up the murder. He never stops mourning Dam-i or resenting his father. He goes off to study in Ming, and as fate would have it, he becomes Dam-i's tutor upon his return. Though the appointment occurs because of evil machinations by her Grandfather, Jung Ji-un soon adapts to the role and quickly falls head over heels for Dam-i, now Crown Prince Dam-i. She knows immediately that he is her childhood love. He does not—and cannot—know that the crown prince is the girl he loved in his youth. Interestingly, there is no nod to homophobia in this show: Jung Ji-un loves the person he loves, period.

The second young man is Jung Ji-un's best friend, Prince Lee Hyun. He learned of Dam-i's secret at the outset of the transition and was by her side over the 10 years of the masquerade, watching her suffer through living a life that wasn't hers. He swore to himself that he would help her. At one point in the show, he reminisces that he used to read to her every night to help her sleep, noting that she loved books and had nightmares. Prince Hyun is the most politically savvy of the three, possibly because he has a terribly conniving brother and always had to manage his intrusive ways. The men are never rivals, because Prince Hyun has always known there was no possible future in which he could be with Dam-i and that she only has eyes for Jung Ji-un.

These three people, Dam-i as Crown Prince Dam-i, Prince Hyun, and Jung Ji-un, are the moral center of the show. Each has strong values and is willing to die for them. Their great affection for one another anchors them through the hardships they face.

Versus the Death Machine

Her grandfather is as thoroughly evil as any villain ever depicted on television. Through his conniving he dethroned one brother and replaced him with his son-in-law, Dam-i's father. The grandfather will kill anyone who is in the way of his chosen puppet king. This *modus operandi* resembles that of the infamous Boss Hague in Jersey City, New Jersey, who would first try to buy people off, then threaten them, and then, if those tactics didn't work, move in for the kill. I don't know how literal the move to kill was in the case of Boss Hague, but in the grandfather's case it was quite literal, and everybody knew it. When Dam-i's father seeks to escape his puppet role, the grandfather poisons him. Thus, Crown Prince

Dam-i eventually becomes king, and the stage is set for a fight to the death between the grandfather and her. The outcome will determine what kind of world will exist for so many others: a world that permits abusive and absolute power over the people or one in which power is modulated by a moral code.

The Arc of the Moral Universe

Reverend Dr. Martin Luther King Jr. said, "The arc of the moral universe is long but it bends toward justice."[4] Unitarian minister Theodore Parker put this idea forward in an 1853 sermon:

> I do not pretend to understand the moral universe; the arc is a long one, my eye reaches but little ways; I cannot calculate the curve and complete the figure by the experience of sight; I can divine it by conscience. And from what I see I am sure it bends towards justice.[5]

Parker was a leading abolitionist and women's rights advocate. He had a sense of how the world worked on these deep problems, which gave him the confidence to say that. He could see, with his own eyes, the ways in which the hard-fought movement against slavery was changing the landscape—fugitive slaves came to find a well-worn path to freedom, while slave catchers met staunch resistance. One of my favorite monuments is the "Jerry Rescue," which commemorates an 1851 event in Syracuse, New York, when slave catchers tried to take a fugitive back to slavery. A crowd, assembled there for an anti-slavery convention, rallied to Jerry's defense, freed him from prison, and spirited him away to Canada. The 1851 rescue, among many other events, would have been part of what Reverend Parker had seen.[6]

Getting to that point in the fight against slavery was very difficult, but they did get there and went even further: slavery was abolished. We have been fighting since to make the United States a place of true equality. We have not gotten there yet, but we can see that things are different and can therefore imagine how much better they might be if we persevere. That is the evidence of the arc of the moral universe bending toward justice.

But why "the *moral* universe"?

In 2006, the Reverend Susan Manker-Seale gave a sermon on the moral arc of the universe bending toward justice.[7] In that sermon she pointed out that the politics of the day were giving the word "moral" a bad reputation:

> In these post-Moral Majority years, the word "moral" dances on the boundary of bad words. It really isn't. Its definition is "of or concerned with the judgment of the goodness or badness of human action and character" (*The Am. Heritage Dictionary*). I think that the description of our moral universe as having a long arc pertains to the fact that history has changing definitions of morality. Jesus was a radical who challenged the moral state of his society, as did [Reverend Theodore] Parker, [Susan B.] Anthony, [Mahatma] Gandhi, [Rosa] Parks and [Martin Luther] King [Jr.]. Time shows that moral values change as we learn more about each other and learn to empathize with each other, to grow from strangers to friends to considering such concepts as the true brotherhood or sisterhood of all humanity, the global community, and the interconnected web of which we are all a part. These concepts lead us to confront what moral behavior really means and to consider where justice lies within our own actions.[8]

Churches, she told her listeners, help their members find and act on the moral issues of their times. She continued:

> I think that Parker and King have given us clues to that journey: Parker said, "Never violate the sacredness of your individual self-respect." King said, "Injustice anywhere is a threat to

justice everywhere" (Birmingham Jail, 4/16/63). Put those two together and we have a simple roadmap. Respect yourself and others, and fight against injustice.[9]

Thus, the "moral" universe is the universe of beliefs we hold, and this is constantly shifting, though not evenly across the globe. One of the injustices at the center of *The King's Affection* is the inferior status of girls. Despite centuries of struggle—it was an issue championed by Parker and King, among many others—women still lag behind men in social standing, economic power, and political leadership. In some places, even their existence is questioned, as it was for Dam-i.

A 2023 article in *The New York Times* shared the story of Sunil Jaglan, a champion for women's rights in India. It noted:

> When the nurse stepped out of the delivery room, her face turned somber as she approached with a baby in her arms wrapped in a blanket. Her voice dropped to a hush, almost like she was ashamed, as she announced to the family: "It is a daughter."
>
> Nothing about the nurse's negative demeanor surprised Sunil Jaglan, the newborn's father. Growing up in the northern Indian state of Haryana, he was accustomed to parents' strong preference for having sons over daughters.
>
> But something within him snapped, he said, when he offered the nurse money as a thank you gesture, and she refused because she had not handed over a boy.
>
> "Are you also ashamed of yourself?" Mr. Jaglan recently remembered asking the nurse when his daughter was born. . . .
>
> That episode transformed him into an unlikely champion of women's rights in a deeply patriarchal society. He turned the nurse's four words, uttered almost as a curse—"It is a daughter"—into a slogan for a campaign that health officials say is responsible for saving the lives of hundreds of girls in Haryana.[10]

Like Sunil Jaglan, Rosa Parks had a moment when the injustice was just too much and she took a principled stance. This precipitated the 1955 Montgomery Bus Boycott. At the mass meeting on the first day of the boycott, the Reverend Dr. Martin Luther King Jr., said to the crowd:

> And you know, my friends, there comes a time when people get tired of being trampled over by the iron feet of oppression. There comes a time, my friends, when people get tired of being plunged across the abyss of humiliation, where they experience the bleakness of nagging despair. There comes a time when people get tired of being pushed out of the glittering sunlight of life's July and left standing amid the piercing chill of an alpine November. There comes a time when time itself is ready for change.[11]

We can understand that as a moment of grace.

Injustice Anywhere Is a Threat to Justice Everywhere

Crown Prince Dam-i had such a moment of grace during the visit of an envoy from Ming.

> The envoy, born in Joseon, was sold to Ming and became Chief Eunuch. He is enraged at the kingdom of Joseon and takes it out on his hosts. He attacks a serving girl. Failing to achieve her ruin, he attacks Crown Prince Dam-i's court lady, shaming her by cutting off her hair.
>
> Crown Prince Dam-i, Jung Ji-un, and Prince Hyun learn not only that Chief Eunuch is stealing from the emperor of Ching but also that he was traumatized by the experience of being sold to Ming. With a compassionate understanding of the source of

the envoy's anger, Crown Prince Dam-i officially apologizes to him on behalf of the kingdom of Joseon. The envoy is visibly mollified, and as he departs for the return journey to Ming, we see the three partners standing shoulder to shoulder, watching him go. It is their first successful joint effort.

Shortly thereafter, another injustice begins to unfold. Lord Chagun, the crazy uncle of Crown Prince Dam-i and Prince Hyun, becomes enraged when a slave girl's basket spills food on his shoes. Crown Prince Dam-i steps in and calls him to task. Unable to wreak his revenge then, Lord Chagun later snatches the girl, intending to rape her. Again Crown Prince Dam-i steps in. Her uncle will not be mollified and later that day kills the girl. Crown Prince Dam-i working with Prince Hyun and Jung Ji-un, finds the knife he used to commit the murder. She demands that he kneel at the slave's grave to ask forgiveness. Horrified, he obeys her command.

Prince Hyun's brother, Prince Wonsan, who wants the throne back for his side of the family, uses this episode with Lord Chagun as a pretext to unite the Confucian scholars against Crown Prince Dam-i. They claim that Crown Prince Dam-i's actions offended the Confucian class system, posing a threat to the stability of society. Their request that the crown prince be dethroned promises to remove one obstacle in the way of Prince Wonsan's achieving his goal.

When Court Lady Kim and Chief Eunuch Hong, Crown Prince Dam-i's household intimates, ask about her actions toward her uncle, Crown Prince Dam-i responds with a statement that clarifies her moral stance:

> She had her life taken from her because she was of low birth and I had to die because I was born a girl. What makes us any different? If I had turned a blind eye yet again, then for another 10 years—no, until the end of my days—my life would have been

filled with nothing more than meaningless attempts to stay alive. What kind of life would that be? That thought crossed my mind. Pretending not to see and hear things for the sake of keeping my place in the palace? What meaning is there in that? The scholars' reactions prove that the code our people live by has not changed since I was born.

At this point I am reminded of Crown Prince Dam-i's mother's instruction that she not help, care for, or get close to others. Her mother's caution may be understood in two ways. First, if people are close to her, they will discern Crown Prince Dam-i's secret. She is right about this. Second, Crown Prince Dam-i will need to be arrogant and distant to survive the political games at the palace. This concern is, I think, less true. Crown Prince Dam-i is not a very able politician and truly needs the people who are close to her. Her furious attack on Lord Chagun reflects a moral position, but it is not a politically savvy act. Astute politicians would have called a war council of their allies to decide how to move—the need to see the chess board 10 moves out is omnipresent in politics, and Crown Prince Dam-i seems to have none of that skill.[12]

During the obsequies for US President Jimmy Carter, many of the reflections turned on this contradiction as it appeared in his life. He knew the game of politics but was only willing to play it to a limited extent. He pursued his moral commitments in spite of political costs.[13]

It is this contradiction that drives the K-drama's plot twists and turns. Crown Prince Dam-i was dethroned and sent away, then brought back and made king. In the role of king, she dedicated herself to taking down her grandfather's reign of terror. One such act was to bring Shin Young-soo, exiled by her grandfather, back from the countryside. The appointment includes a note from her that says simply, "*Bulbibulmyeong*." Luckily for me, people in the show explain that this is a bird that sits silently for three years, then rises to the sky and pierces the earth with its cry. Shin Young-soo, on his return, says to King Dam-i, "Does that refer to your majesty?" She says nothing. He then says that he won't follow her on the wrong path. She gives him evidence of perfidy in government, and he moves quickly to unearth it and get justice. This sets up the final, fatal confrontation.

As King Dam-i's confrontation with her grandfather escalates, her "I can do it" attitude makes her vulnerable to the "fog of war," which sets in.[14] She says to Jung Ji-un, "I feel as if I'm surrounded by fog. When I run somewhere thinking it's my final destination, I realize that the destination is actually still far away. And when I run with all my might it gets farther away. I have been wandering around to no end. I feel like I have forgotten where I need to go. Will I be able to find my way again? Will the fog ever go away?"

Jung Ji-un, who is wise, sensitive, and a highly trained healer, replies with confidence and kindness in his voice, "Once the rain stops, the sun will shine. Once the fog lifts, the view will become clear. If you have a destination, you will reach it someday. No matter how long it takes."

I sense that, in her confusion, King Dam-i fails to anticipate her grandfather's decision to bring in the private army he'd been building. He knows that she has caught him in his perfidy—poisoning her father and stealing from the government. He needs to destroy her and her allies before she can act against him.

Her team fights valiantly against his army but is defeated. Back against the wall, King Dam-i calmly requests that her grandfather drink tea with her one last time before he kills her. The tea is laced with the same poison her grandfather used to kill her father. Because she drinks first, her grandfather thinks the tea is safe and drinks it. He is furious when he realizes the trick she's played but is, of course, dead before he can act on his rage.

Why didn't Dam-i die? Recapper SailorJumun proposed that the anti-anxiety medicine Jung Ji-un had given her is what saves her, for which we can be very thankful.[15]

The Bend

Dam-i had long committed to taking responsibility for the lie she enacted. In the penultimate scene of the show, she is brought to trial before her dear Hyun, who is now king. The charges state: "Ascending to the throne, while lying about her gender, is equivalent to making a mockery of the officials and the people. This is a serious offense that can weaken ROYAL ORDER, the foundation of the nation."

Shin Young-soo, who is highly esteemed for his learning and probity, steps forward to speak on her behalf. He makes the speech that summarizes the whole moral conflict:

> Based on the ideology of Neo-Confucianism that men and women have different duties, it is clear that what she had done is indeed a serious, unforgivable offense. However, the preceding king did not intend to become the prince years ago and was forced to take the crown prince's place. And upon taking the throne, the preceding king attempted to rule the nation with the highest form of benevolence in history for the better[ment] of the people. Thus, it is unjust to punish the preceding king only based on doctrine and ideology. The preceding king did not make a mockery of the people.

With passion in his voice, Shin Young-soo concludes:

> This only took place because a group of corrupt rebels chased power instead of serving our king. I ask that you punish all of

> your subjects who had turned a blind eye on their corrupt acts before you punish the preceding king.

He then kneels by her side. All the ministers join in the plea for mercy. A flashback shows us Jung Ji-un suggesting *paenghyeong* as a way forward for King Hyun to take. *Paenghyeong* is the act of erasing a life from the official record. In a Neo-Confucian society, *paenghyeong* would be a severe punishment,[16] but in this case it is the opposite. King Hyun pronounces the sentence that "Lee Hwi," her dead brother's name, will be erased from the records and Dam-i left with no name. She is liberated.

Around the Bend

In the final sequence, the show takes us to Arcadia, where Jung Ji-un and Dam-i—now Yeon-seon—are playing at hunting for dinner. As they walk on the shore, they see their friends coming to greet them—King Hyun, Court Lady Kim, Chief Eunuch Hong, and bodyguard Kang Eun-seo, her "home team" during the long battle. We leave them hugging one another as the waves wash upon the shore and the sun sets (Figure 7.1).

What Is a Friend?

The joy of the moment is, I think, meant to be kept in our hearts, to warm us on the long days when the struggle for justice seems all too hard. The arc is long, and we cannot see all the way. We must, as Reverend Parker instructed during the hard fight against slavery, *discern by conscience* that it bends toward justice.

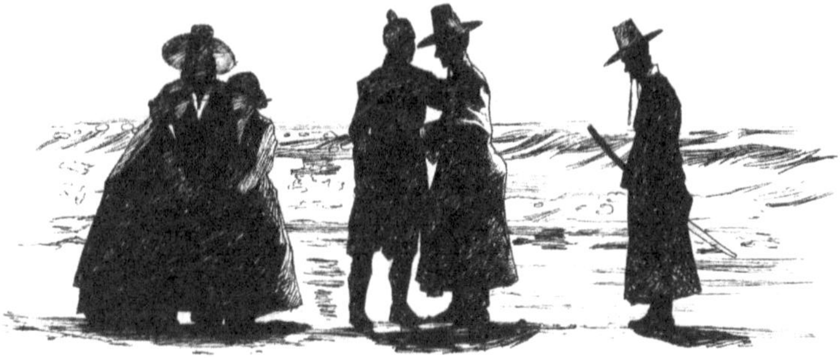

Figure 7.1 On the Beach.
In the final scene of *The King's Affection* the posse reunites on the beach.
Drawing by Mike Malbrough, used with permission.

Why do we keep the love of friends in our heart?

This is not a trivial teaching but perhaps the heart of the matter for the Tao of K-drama. We do not bend the moral arc by ourselves, but in collaboration with others. Some of those by our side become friends.

In his field-building book *Everything in Its Path*, Kai Erikson wrote about the displacement of some towns along Buffalo Creek, which flooded as a result of a mine accident. Homes were washed away, and people lost the commu nities in which they were anchored. Their grief was profound. Erikson, in a brilliant move, did not presume that he knew what they meant when they said "neighbor." Instead, to understand why it hurt so much to be separated from neighbors, he asked, "What is a neighbor?" One man replied, "What is a neighbor? Well, when I went to my neighbor's house on Saturday or Sunday, if I wanted a cup of coffee I never waited until the lady of the house asked me. I just went into the dish cabinet and got me a cup of coffee or a glass of juice just like it was my own home. They come to my house, they done the same. See?"[17]

That exchange comes back to me while studying the Tao of K-drama. In scene after scene, I see evidence of deep friendship. Sometimes it is signaled in the language. In a scene that takes place during childhood, Prince Hyun and Jung Ji-un greet each other. Jung Ji-un's father admonishes him for speaking informally to a prince. Prince Hyun smiles and says that they are friends and he gave Jung Ji-un permission to do so.

One signal of intimacy is the addition of "ah" after a name, as in "Hyun-ah" and "Ji-un-ah." This is often used when slipping out of formal speech forms into *banmal*, or informal speech. The forms of address—like the freedom to have some orange juice—are symbolic of the underlying relationship. These details are not noted in the subtitles and therefore are obscured, at least for English-speaking audiences who lack formal/informal indicators as part of our grammar. I am very grateful for the guidance of Professor Park, who explained these matters to me.

The Neo-Confucians were ambivalent about friendship because it created strong horizontal bonds. *The King's Affection* pays attention to Neo-Confucian rules of society—we see numerous episodes of people studying the texts. A key scene between Jung Ji-un and Crown Prince Dam-i involves him challenging her to answer a question he poses about the lotus. The question alludes to her grandfather's dirty politics. The correct answer, which she misses, is that the lotus grows in mud but is not dirty. This teaching is an act of friendship offered to protect her from her grandfather's evil. It illustrates what the Neo-Confucians feared, which is the subversive side of friendship that could disrupt the social order—friends are chosen, good friends support one's moral life, and friends offer freedom of choice because they are not fixed in the hierarchy.

Given her grandfather's complete abandonment of the tenets of Neo-Confucianism—the reciprocity between subjects and rulers—friendship becomes the source of moral inspiration and social power needed to right the ship. Norman Kutcher, in an illuminating paper on Neo-Confucian views of friendship, observes that friendships are based on shared struggles and that such friendships ought to be cherished for life.[18] A beautiful article in *The New York Times* echoed that sentiment in describing the way in which an immigrant woman's kindness to a young man finding his way in the city created a lifelong friendship. Later in life, when the woman was older and weaker, her young friend was able to repay her kindness, saving her bar and making her a lifelong employee so that she would have income, health care benefits, and a place of welcome.[19]

It is the passion of friendship, what the recappers call "bromance," and the closeness of friendship, what people refer to as "the brother from another mother," that is celebrated in K-drama. In *The King's Affection*, we see the sharp contrast between the relationships formed by expediency and intimidation—indeed, everything the grandfather touches—and true friendship based on moral values and love.

But perhaps the most unexpected story of friendship and its link to moral values is that of Jung Seok-jo, Jung Ji-un's father, the man who assassinated Dam-i's brother. Jung Seok-jo came of age with Yoon Hyeong-seol, who is the protector of Crown Prince Dam-i. Yoon Hyeong-seol confronts Jung Seok-jo on several occasions. At first Jung Seok-jo counters that he had no choice—the path he is on is the only one that was offered to him. Unlike Dam-i—who also had no choice—he does not follow this assertion with acknowledgment that he will one day face judgment.

Then Jung Seok-jo is sent to chase down Yoon Hyeong-seol, who has stolen information on the grandfather's illicit schemes. When they catch up with Yoon Hyeong-seol, Jung Seok-jo's archers unleash a flight of arrows. Jung Seok-jo screams, "NOOOOO!" He holds Yoon Hyeong-seol as he lies dying and remembers the friendship and love they shared as youths. While his love for his son and awareness that his son loves a good woman—for he is another one who knows King Dam-i is a woman—have been causing him to waver in his loyalty to the grandfather, it is Yoon Hyeong-seol's death that moves him to Dam-i's side.

What is a friend? I believe that friendship is walking side by side on the moral path—this is the true source of love.

8

Peace Between the Nations

Captain Ri Crosses the Line

> Peace, to have meaning for many who have known only suffering in both peace and war, must be translated into bread or rice, shelter, health, and education, as well as freedom and human dignity—a steadily better life.
>
> —Ralph Bunche

> He: "I did not go to the south: you came to the north."
> She, in English: "*N-n-n-north Korea*?"
>
> —Captain Ri and Yoon Se-ri, *Crash Landing on You*

> When the war is won,
> Treat it as you would a funeral.
>
> —*The Tao*, No. 31

There is a debate about how many plot lines there are in fiction.[1] Mary Morris commented:

> John Gardner once said that there are only two plots in all of literature: you go on a journey, or the stranger comes to town.
>
> Since women, for so many years, were denied the journey, we were left with only one plot to our lives—to await the stranger. Indeed, there is no picaresque tradition among women who are novelists. Women's literature, from Austen to Woolf, is

> mostly about waiting, usually for love. Denied the freedom to roam outside themselves, women turned inward, into their emotions.[2]

In the 21st-century story *Crash Landing on You*, known to its fans as CLOY, it is a woman who goes on a journey. Paragliding heroine Yoon Se-ri gets caught in a tornado and is blown into the demilitarized zone (DMZ), the most heavily mined and monitored place in the world and the strip of land that separates North and South Korea (Figure 8.1). She lands in a tree. Our hero, the North Korean officer, Ri Jeong-hyeok, barks at her to get down out of the tree. She obeys, falling into his arms. She notices his uniform and thinks it must be that he is escaping from North Korea, or possibly that he's a spy on a mission. He breaks into these musings to set the record straight. "I did not go to the south: you came to the north."

She sputters in English, "North Korea?"[3]

She offers to run home quietly and quickly. He makes it clear that that is not an option.

As the extent of her troubles dawns on Yoon Se-ri, Ri Jeong-hyeok remains impassive, thinking he has control. But no, he is wrong; things are about to spiral for both of them. By the time he drags her off the street of the North Korean village where he lives, it is clear that "We have a situation here!"[4]

Georges Polti, author of *Thirty-Six Dramatic Situations*, didn't buy Gardner's "two plots" idea.[5] He believed there could be multiple plots in any given show: the main plot might be one situation, but a subplot could be a different one. That is certainly the case in *Crash Landing on You.*

Here are some of the plots in CLOY, along with the names they have in Polti's system. Yoon Se-ri falls into the arms of the upstanding Ri Jeong-hyeok, who takes responsibility for her deliverance (Polti 2: Deliverance). In addition, the show works from a premise of "equal-opportunity evil." A North Korean criminal, Cho

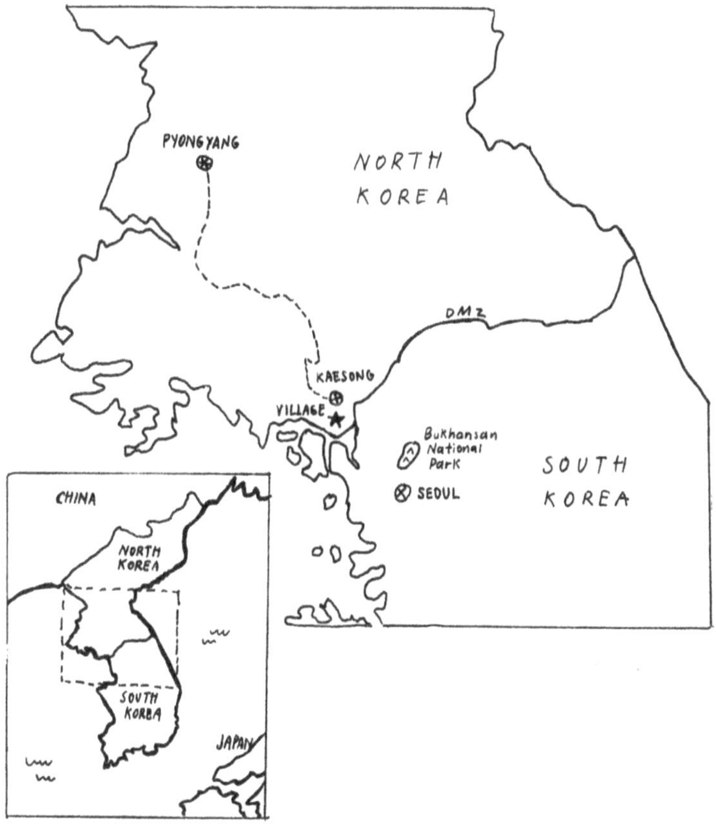

Figure 8.1 Map of Korea.
Map created by Laura Van Vleet and Aya Maruyama and used with permission.

Cheol-gang, wants to destroy Ri Jeong-hyeok's family and sees the capture of Yoon Se-ri as the quickest way to do this (Polti 3: Crime Pursued by Vengeance). Yoon Se-ri's older brother wants her to disappear so that he can control the family business. Killing her is one easy way to do this, and he is urged on by his wife, a real Lady MacBeth (Polti 14: Rivalry of Kinsmen). Also, because Yoon Se-ri is her father's love child, her stepmother wants her out, though later the stepmother comes to regret her hatred and murderous impulse (Polti 13: Enmity of Kinsmen). Finally, Yoon Se-ri and Captain Ri are from two countries with absolute separation, so they face Polti's No. 28, Obstacles to Love. There are more subplots, but we'll stop here.

This sprawling drama is what powers us through the 16 episodes and shows individualistic Americans how community works. The main plot line of *Crash Landing on You* is Deliverance: Ri Jeong-hyeok must deliver Yoon Se-ri back to South Korea. The clash of the impenetrable border and the yearning of their love gives the plot its particular flavor, for her deliverance means they will never see each other again. In this bittersweet story, the reward for success is loss of the beloved. Other dramatists have explored this situation, including J. M. Barrie in *Admiral Crichton* and Richard Rodgers in *No Strings*. In each case, the dramatists used the storyline to critique division: Korea's partition in *Crash Landing on You*, the British class system in *Admiral Crichton*, and racial prejudice in *No Strings*.

Our hero, Ri Jeong-hyeok—handsome, talented, and born to a high-ranking father who was able to send him to Switzerland to study piano—was a golden child of North Korea. But his glamorous life ended abruptly with the death of his older brother. He returned immediately to North Korea and stepped into his brother's military career. Ri Jeong-hyeok is a highly moral man of action who has withdrawn on an emotional level; he is no longer the open, smiling youth we glimpse in flashbacks. His mother is anguished by her son's lack of connection with others.

Yoon Se-ri has scars of her own left by childhood traumas. She was taken from her biological mother to be raised by her father and his family. Because her existence is proof of her father's infidelity, her stepmother wants nothing to do with her and lets her sons pick on her. One day her stepmother abandons Yoon Se-ri on a beach, where the poor child counts over and over, sure her stepmother will return. Instead, Yoon Se-ri is saved by strangers and lives with the pain of her stepmother's abandonment. Fear of abandonment sets the tone for Yoon Se-ri's life.

In my experience as a psychiatrist, loss of trust is the core harm resulting from trauma of any kind. It fosters fear and drives a persistent need to feel safe. This has a profound effect on decision-making. Rather than thinking widely and unselfishly about the potential outcomes of any situation, the traumatized person is likely to place preservation of self first, even at the expense of others. In *Crash Landing on You,* we see this dynamic at play on Christmas Eve at Yoon Se-ri's fashion company. She is aware of the needs of her employees, yet she sniffs disdainfully at them and makes her team continue working. The contrast between the office atmosphere inside and the snowfall and merry revelers outside reminds us of Scrooge and *The Christmas Carol.*

Stranger Danger

Crash Landing on You plays Yoon Se-ri's arrival in North Korea as a lighthearted comedy of errors that keeps us laughing until reality hits.

> Fight, freeze, or flight is the classic stress response. Yoon Se-ri sees herself as a fast runner and she's dressed in high-quality athleisure wear.[6] She runs from Captain Ri Jeong-hyeok. He goes after her. She has managed to cross a stream. While on the opposite bank, he steps on a landmine. When she hears the telltale click of the detonator, she taunts him. He begs her to leave his walkie-talkie, which she places on a rock midstream. Then she bolts off. He calls after her, "The path will divide—go to the right and you'll be in your country."

On the back of her jumpsuit is emblazoned the name of her company: Seri's Choice. The name, we learn, is inspired by a family story about the choice she made at her first birthday party, an important occasion in South Korea. My Korean-language textbook provides this explanation of that event, known as 돌 (*dol*):

> An interesting tradition of 돌 is 돌잡이. Items such as money, rice, books, pencils, thread, a microphone, and so on are arranged on a table for the baby to pick up. It is believed that the item which the baby picks foretells the baby's future. Money and rice are interpreted as symbols of a wealthy life, books and pencils as academic success, thread as a long and healthy life, and the microphone as a promising career in the entertainment business.[7]

At her 돌, Yoon Se-ri was presented with a lavish table of choices but instead chose her father's hand. The guests interpreted this as particularly auspicious.

Yoon Se-ri notes, in a voiceover, that she has always relied on her ability to choose, which she credits for her fabulous success in building a fashion company. So, when she arrives at the fork in the road Ri Jeong-hyeok told her she'd find, she debates what to do. Should she heed the handsome officer's advice and go to the right? Or was he trying to trick her? She concludes he was being devious and heads left.

Captain Ri, meanwhile, has to be liberated from the landmine. One of his men, Kim Kwang-beom, arrives shortly after Yoon Se-ri scampers off. When Captain Ri asks if he knows how to defuse a mine, Kim Kwang-beom replies he has only defused a mine once during his training. Captain Ri, like a helicopter mom, keeps asking nervous questions and Kim Kwang-beom gives him the "give me a break" look as he holds up the pin.

Freed, Captain Ri orders his squad of four men to catch Yoon Se-ri as she races through the minefields. Master Sergeant Pyo Chi-soo, having convinced some fellow soldiers to join him in having some "medicine," wakes up with a terrible hangover

> and fails to understand Captain Ri's order to capture Yoon Se-ri without harming her. He chases after her, firing off shots, but can't shoot straight. Convinced that they mean to harm her, Yoon Se-ri runs faster.
>
> Captain Ri and Kim Kwang-beom reach Master Sergeant Pyo Chi-soo just as Yoon Se-ri makes it through a minefield and reaches a fence. A downed tree makes it possible for her to get to the other side. They all yell at her not to cross. Determined to escape her pursuers and reach safety, Yoon Se-ri jumps over the fence . . . into North Korea!
>
> Up in a guard tower, Sergeant Kim Joo-meok should have seen Yoon Se-ri lope by, but he was watching a forbidden South Korean drama, *Stairway to Heaven*. And Geum Eun-dong, the homesick youngest member of Captain Ri's group and the last line of defense against the intruder from the south, is too busy crying over a letter from his mom to see Yoon Se-ri speeding past.

Recapper LollyPip notes, "[The] squad are flat-out adorable, reminding me of hapless little ducklings as they stumble around following their not-much-more savvy mama duck. I hope that they do find Se-ri, and that they form a weird little family, because I think Se-ri could use some better 'brothers' even if they are the enemy."[8]

The "adorable ducklings" did not act as if they were in the most heavily fortified place in the world. As in many high-anxiety situations, most of the time nothing happens. The quiet lulls people into believing it will stay that way, and they let down their guard. And then *CRASH*—Yoon Se-ri landed on them.

> Eventually, Yoon Se-ri arrives in a forest and thrashes around, falling, getting lost, but still confident that she will get somewhere. Eventually, she emerges on a hillside. A man with an ox cart passes her and she learns he doesn't have a cell phone. Women gather around to get eggs. The street lights come on and

a big sign announces that the great leader is always with us. Yoon Se-ri, deep in shock, is suddenly blinded by the headlights of a jeep. She is pulled into the yard of a house, just as Captain Ri's enemy, the terrible Cho Cheol-gang, drives by.

Inside the yard, with the gate safely closed, she again faces Captain Ri.

She thinks, "I can charm him."

He thinks, "Should I kill her?"

They are no longer in the DMZ but the horrors of the unfinished Korean War stand between them.

The Korean War

In 1910, Korea was annexed by Japan and was considered part of its empire until August 1945, when Japan surrendered to the Allied forces. Although freed of colonial occupation, Korea's troubles continued as the Cold War between capitalism and socialism took center stage.

The US administration was aware that communism had gained an important toehold in Korea during the struggle against Japanese colonialism. Concerned that the Soviet Union was encroaching on Korea from the north, US forces were deployed to the region to preemptively limit the Soviet advance. This action was accompanied by a US declaration that Korea would be divided at the 38th parallel.[9] Following the Soviet troop withdrawal in 1948, Korean communists, led by Kim Il Sung and his fellow anti-Japanese guerillas, emerged as the leaders in the north. The US, echoing the Japanese occupiers' claim that they were guiding Korea into the future, installed a series of hand-picked, anti-communist leaders in the south. The US maintained massive military forces in the region and funneled billions in aid to keep the south "safe for democracy." Notably, the US did not install a democracy.

Reunification was the objective of leaders on both sides of the 38th parallel. Military forays across this demarcation escalated for several years, resulting in the outbreak of the war in June 1950. The United Nations was authorized by Security Council Resolution 82 to send armed forces to oppose North Korea's troops. In the first phase of the war, Kim Il Sung's troops pushed rapidly south but failed to push the UN forces off the peninsula. Joint UN and US forces pushed back, taking the war to the north, where they followed Kim Il Sung's troops deep into the mountain fastness. At that point, UN and US forces, unfamiliar with the terrain, were easy pickings for the local troops and suffered massive losses. China came into the war on the side of North Korea and together they pushed the UN and US forces south of the 38th parallel.

What happened then, in my view, was a bitter reprisal by the US administration for the humiliation of both the drive south and the bitter defeat they'd suffered in the north. US forces launched airstrikes that wiped out every city, town, and village in the north, leaving the people huddling in caves. Mao Tse-tung's son, Mao Anying, was killed during one of the airstrikes.

Historians estimate that between three and four million Koreans died, most of them civilians.[10] Jeremy Kumarov, in a detailed analysis of the war and its consequences, wrote:

> Apart from the question of whether the Korean War was necessary, the horrible human cost of the war marks it as one of the worst ever fought. Saint Augustine of Hippo (354–430 CE) considered war a crime if it was fought with "malicious intent to destroy, a desire to dominate with fierce hatred and furious vengeance," which was clearly the case for Korea. While 36,574 Americans died, three to four million Koreans lost their lives as a result of the war, including one out of every nine North Koreans, according to a UN estimate. In addition, six to seven million Koreans were rendered refugees and over 8,500 factories, 5,000 schools, 1,000 hospitals, and 600,000 homes were destroyed.[11]

It is important to add that 100,000 children were orphaned. Orphans are stigmatized in Korea, and many Korean babies, unable to be adopted in their own country, were adopted abroad.[12]

James I. Matray wrote of the war:

> An armistice ended fighting in Korea on July 27, 1953. Since then, Koreans have seen the war as the second-greatest tragedy in their recent history after Japanese colonial rule. Not only did it cause devastation and three million deaths, it also confirmed the division of a homogeneous society after thirteen centuries of unity. The partition permanently separated millions of families. Meanwhile, US wartime spending jump-started Japan's economy, which led to its emergence as a global power. Koreans, on the other hand, had to endure the living tragedy of yearning for reunification. As we know all too well, diplomatic tension and military clashes along the demilitarized zone continue and are considered by many a threat far beyond the region.[13]

From "Enemies" to Buddies

The history of the war and the development of the two countries since then have set up for Westerners the idea of a "failed" North Korea and a "successful" South Korea. CLOY is not telling exactly that story. When I taught this K-drama to a class at The New School, they used Airtable to make a detailed database of every scene in the show. Each student took an aspect of the drama and developed it into a paper, and all of these papers were collected in our book, *One Step Can't Hurt: Situation Analysis through the Lens of K-Drama.*[14] As I noted in Chapter 1, Audrey Jenkins was interested in a concept she called "care" and looked at the many ways in which large and small acts of care and "anti-care" were demonstrated. The story presented care and anti-care in both North and South Korea but distributed them differently. In this diagram from Jenkins's paper, we can see the contrast that she observed (Figure 8.2).

Both countries had infrastructures of care, but the two were remarkably different. In North Korea, care was manifested in the community and the communal space, but the country had spotty electricity and limited medical resources. In South Korea, care was manifested as part of the superstructure of social institutions and organizations, but social isolation and family abuse undermined Yoon Se-ri's individual well-being.

The many ways in which CLOY distributed good and evil on both sides of the DMZ contributed to an equilibrium between the two firmly divided countries. As the characters experienced these infrastructures of care, they could let go of stigmatizing assumptions and engage as human beings. This is, of course, the foundational concept of the people-to-people exchanges that have become extremely important in our embattled world. The honesty and goodwill of the unfolding encounter is what will save Yoon Se-ri and her new "family."

> The morning after Yoon Se-ri's unexpected arrival, Captain Ri makes her breakfast. She is afraid of being poisoned and says it is the custom in South Korea for the host to taste the food first. He shakes his head at her. Then Master Sergeant Pyo Chi-soo, who had been too drunk to follow orders or shoot straight, arrives at the house. He is excited because an unidentified young woman was found dead by the highway. He is convinced this must be the woman they lost the day before. Master Sergeant Pyo Chi-soo chatters on about the relief he feels: homesick Geum Eun-dong won't be discharged, Sergeant Kim Joo-meok won't be disciplined for leaving his post to watch K-drama, and he won't be admonished for having a glass of wine—no big deal, anyway. Yoon Se-ri comes out of the house and overhears Master Sergeant Pyo Chi-soo while Captain Ri, who sees her standing there, shakes his head in disbelief. Yoon Se-ri confronts Master Sergeant

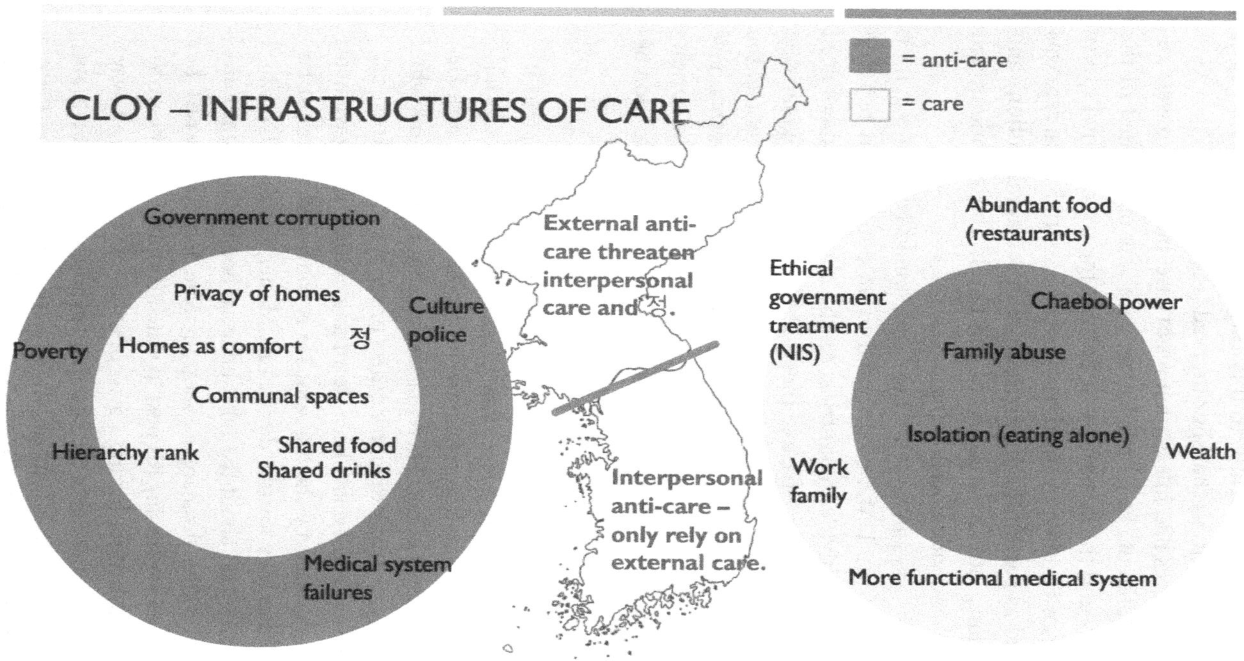

Figure 8.2 Infrastructure of Care in *Crash Landing on You.*
This diagram compares the representation of caring acts in the two countries, North Korea on the left and South Korea on the right.
Created by Audrey A. Jenkins, used with permission.

Master Sergeant Pyo Chi-soo and they have the first of many arguments. The others arrive believing the story that the dead woman is the person they failed to catch the day before. They are quickly disabused of that idea.

Yoon Se-ri, with the knowledge she overheard from Master Sergeant Pyo Chi-soo, quickly identifies who's who in the crew. She makes friends with Sergeant Kim Joo-meok, asking him which K-drama he was watching. She lets him know that the stars are friends of hers. Grinning, he exclaims, "Really?"

Sergeant Kim Joo-meok has a special place in the hearts of non-Koreans who love K-drama: he is so entranced by a show that he messes up his job, interprets every situation through the lens of something he saw in a show, and feels confident that he knows South Korea because, after all, he has seen K-drama.[15]

Sergeant Kim Joo-meok is chastised for letting his guard down and immediately apologizes, but round 1 goes to Yoon Se-ri. She points out that if she is discovered, they will all be in trouble. Master Sergeant Pyo Chi-soo proposes killing her, because she might be a spy. This is dismissed and soon they start to like one another. Their focus shifts from fears she is a spy to plotting how to get her out of North Korea.

The first crisis to hit this new "family" is a surprise house inspection by the fearsome Cho Cheol-gang. As soon as they learn about it, the squad calls Captain Ri, who is in Pyongyang. Yoon Se-ri is trembling as Cho Cheol-gang holds a gun to her head when Captain Ri arrives in a special car that awes the villagers. He strides up and announces, "Would you take the gun away from my fiancée's head?"

This works.

The next day the squad grabs Captain Ri to get the story. Captain Ri says, "I just introduced her to them and said I was tired and it was time to go to sleep. They said OK."

Master Sergeant Pyo Chi-soo digs: "How did you introduce her?"

Captain Ri owns up: "I said she was my fiancée."

Master Sergeant Pyo Chi-soo is somewhat incredulous and says, "Really?"

Captain Ri is taken aback. He says, "There was no other way—I guess you could call it a disguise tactic."

At this the squad glows at him and Master Sergeant Pyo Chi-soo says sagely, "We shouldn't have been worried then. We didn't know you could lie so well."

Captain Ri starts to defend his honor but Sergeant Kim Joo-meok breaks in, saying, "I've seen scenes like this in South Korean dramas when the characters are hiding and about to be caught."

Master Sergeant Pyo Chi-soo asks, "Then what happens?"

Sergeant Kim Joo-meok explains, "The man and the woman hug each other or kiss each other."

Put off by this idea, Master Sergeant Pyo Chi-soo wonders why they do that.

"That's the South Korean way to avert crises," Sergeant Kim Joo-meok explains, happy to share his insider knowledge.

Geum Eun-dong wonders what happens after that.

"Yaaah," says Sergeant Kim Joo-meok, really warming to his task. "The dramas get more interesting because the two spend the night together."

At that, they all look at Captain Ri, and Kim Kwang-beom points out that Captain Ri didn't come back the night before. Captain Ri tries to defend himself, saying, "Well, we weren't really together. I slept in my room and she slept on the floor in the other room. We were not together."

But Sergeant Kim Joo-meok finds that to be quibbling. "In the shows they all fall in love. One hundred percent. I haven't seen any drama characters that don't fall in love in that situation," he says.

At this point Captain Ri feels he has to take control. He leans forward, squeezes Sergeant Kim Joo-meok's leg in warning, and says, "Sergeant Kim, are you showing off that you've seen a lot of dramas?"

The hilarity of the interchange might distract from the seriousness of the message. In undertaking the task of protecting an illegal immigrant, Captain Ri's rigid, by-the-book style is not going to work. He has to respond in the moment, using what tools he can, including "disguise tactics" and other lies—and even kissing: Sergeant Kim Joo-meok's "South Korean evasion" tip will turn out to be quite useful. That Captain Ri and Yoon Se-ri will fall in love—and maybe already have—is a foregone conclusion. Between experiencing love and evil, Captain Ri will grow and change, learning to lean on his squad through it all.

The strength of his leadership turns out to be his ability to adapt and improvise, key attributes for surviving the "fog of war," per Schmitt and Klein.[16] The fog of war is more extreme than the confusion of daily life—after all, in war people are trying to kill one another. But the image is very useful in considering *Crash Landing on You* because everyone's life is at risk: the squad's because they're harboring a South Korean, thus breaking military discipline, and Yoon Se-ri's because she's a South Korean in North Korea. And that is not all: Cho Cheol-gang is gunning for Captain Ri and his family, while Yoon Se-ri's older brother wants to take her out. In this set of complex situations, our protagonists must continually adjust, improvise, and adapt as events unfold and new threats are uncovered.

The Paradox of Powerlessness

Yoon Se-ri has to make adjustments too. That her choice of taking the left branch of the path was so wrong does not stop her from thinking she can seize control. Her fundamental belief is that she can—and must—rely only on herself.

She has the upper hand after overhearing the squad admit that they screwed up, and she recognizes that they share her danger. Her confidence grows when she completely wins over Sergeant Kim Joo-meok by telling him she knows the star of *Stairway to Heaven*. For a moment, they seem under her command as they deliberate how to get her out of North Korea. Of course—this being K-drama—nothing is going to be simple. But Yoon Se-ri has confidence in her powers of manipulation. It takes a whole Lemony-Snicket series of events to strip her of that confidence.

At one point, she finds herself lost in a North Korean market at dusk, unsure of where she is or how to get back to Captain Ri's house. She stands in the marketplace, frozen with fear, remembering the terrible night on the beach, waiting for her stepmother's return, and counting.

The Korean language has two counting systems, one called Native Korean numbers and the other called Sino-Korean numbers. It's a mix-and-match system, in which one set is used for some things and the other for other things. For example, in telling time, Native Korean numbers are used for the hours and Sino-Korean for the minutes. In Yoon Se-ri's memory, she as a child is counting in Native Korean numbers. As a lost adult, she starts counting in Sino-Korean numbers. The scene moves back and forth between the two.[17]

Captain Ri arrives, unsure how to find her in the maze of stalls and crowd of people. He buys a scented candle and holds it aloft for her to see. Seeing the light, she begins to move. The camera follows the slow motion of her feet as she moves toward him, step by tiny step. Eventually she stands in front of him, the candle's glow reflected in her face. The song *Flower*, sung by Yoon Mi-rae, is playing in the background. The words tell us, "I am worried about you" and "I'll always be by your side."

"By my side" is a Korean expression fraught with meaning. I was shocked when I realized that it was the simple preposition 옆에 (beside) that is carrying the promise of solidarity through thick and thin. Arriving in a moment when Yoon Se-ri knows she is not in control, Captain Ri offers her reliable and loving companionship, something she has not known before. She now has two experiences, one of protecting herself and the other of being protected. A new flexibility enters her life. Paradoxically, it was when she lost control that she gained some safety in the life-threatening situation.[18]

Parting Is Such Sweet Sorrow

After a number of false starts, Captain Ri finds a way to smuggle Yoon Se-ri out of the country. He has to take her through the northern sector of the DMZ to the interior line of division. On the other side of that line she will meet South Korean patrols. They walk through the night, Captain Ri taking the "longest way round" to prolong their time together. Finally, she crosses the line. He realizes he can't let her go without a final kiss. He rationalizes to himself, "One step can't hurt." He steps over the line, grabs Yoon Se-ri, and gives her a kiss. It is wonderful.

Band of Brothers and One Sister

In Episode 13, we witness more of the arc of relationship building in the group. Captain Ri is in Seoul to catch Cho Cheol-gang, who wants to capture Yoon Se-ri to complete his destruction of Ri's family. Captain Ri's father has sent his son's squad plus the eavesdropper Jung Man-beok, known as "the Rat," to bring him safely back to North Korea. The men have gathered at Yoon Se-ri's apartment to celebrate her birthday, which, as the despised love child, is painful for her, and she runs out of the house crying. Captain Ri follows and comforts her. Back at the house, the men share their shock. Even Master Sergeant Pyo Chi-soo admits his worry for her: "Even when I said I would bury her, she didn't cry."

Of course, Master Sergeant Pyo Chi-soo denies any feelings for her when she returns.

The group sings the North Korean happy birthday song to her, which she never expected to hear. And they light candles, which they have not done before. She explains that now all should make a wish, which they close their eyes and do. Then they all join in to blow out the candles.

I've never seen this kind of collective wish making before and have to say, if you're not crying by then, you are really hard-hearted. But have no fear—the episode has more to offer.

The squad was smuggled into South Korea as part of a sports team. They are due to leave, but all refuse out of love for Yoon Se-ri and Captain Ri. Instead, they stay to fight the enemies. The first encounter is with Cho Cheol-gang's thugs. Se-ri's family has lured her to the Yoon family home, plotting to kill her on the way. She drives into a section of road that is deserted and a series of cars block her way. Men armed with sticks come toward her car, not expecting the doors to open and the squad to emerge. A fight ensues. At one point Se-ri asks in a terrified voice, "Are you OK?"

Sergeant Kim Joo-meok answers merrily, "Don't worry! We're from the special forces!"

The enemy is completely defeated.

A Few Words about the Soundtrack

As I've noted, every K-drama has a soundtrack. It is a remarkable thing, and perhaps the reason soundtracks are making a comeback in US films.[19] One of the best original soundtracks, in my opinion, is the one for *Crash Landing on You.* The show was well funded and was able to hire the outstanding composer Nam Hye-seung to do the soundtrack. She and her colleagues wrote many pieces, which were performed by top musicians. Wikipedia has entries for every K-drama, and composers and musicians are typically well documented. The entry for CLOY includes a very unusual feature, the chart performance of the main songs, which is shown in Table 8.1.[20]

Table 8.1 Chart Position of Songs from the *Crash Landing on You* Original Soundtrack

		Peak Positions	
Song Title	**Artist**	**KOR Gaon**	**KOR Hot**
But It's Destiny	10 cm	108	72
Flower	Yoon Mi-rae	22	20
Sunset	Davichi	47	32
Here I Am Again	Baek Ye-rin	4	6
Someday	Kim Jae-hwan	18	17
Photo of My Mind	Song Ga-in	35	31
The Hill of Yearning	April 2	187	—
All of My Days	Sejeong	50	31
Let Us Go	Crush	3	7
Give You My Heart	IU	1	3

Source: Adapted from Wikipedia, *Crash Landing on You.*

CLOY's expansive musical buffet can arouse a full array of feelings, while keeping us centered in the longing for togetherness that is the hallmark of the show. As my personal favorite of the chart toppers, "Hill of Yearning," puts it,

> The song of you and I
> Calls out . . .
> Are you listening?[21]

There is a second tier of songs not included in the chart but possibly even more important to the subtlety of the show. These are the songs that highlight specific characters or specific relationships.

The jaunty "Like You" depicts the delight of Yoon Se-ri and Captain Ri's emerging affection. The slightly discordant "Chi Soo and Seri" captures the contentious relationship they have. "Picnic" takes us away from daily life, but with the undercurrent of the parting that is to follow the outing.

Perhaps the most important song is one purportedly written by Captain Ri, called "Song for My Brother." Yoon Se-ri heard this song in the depths of her suicidal mission in Switzerland and it distracted her and gave her a certain hope. She remembers it precisely and plays it for all the musicians she meets, hoping to find someone who knows it. Eventually she plays it for Captain Ri, who plays it back to her.

In this show, Nam Hye Seung uses chilly Icelandic rock music for painful scenes. The end of *Crash Landing on You* is much more difficult than that of *Romance Is a Bonus Book*: our lovers have organized a way to meet in Switzerland for two weeks a year. But I was watching the show during COVID, when North Korea had closed its borders completely. In our reality, even that small bit of comfort would have been snatched from them. The song playing at the end is called "Sigriswil," which is the name of a bridge in Switzerland. The lyrics are in English and talk about "the times we had back in the day." The song's chilly, ethereal tones are insubstantial in a way that is disconcerting, even without COVID. It is profound to watch the show come to a close, and it perhaps explains the joy experienced worldwide after the stars, Hyun Bin and Son Ye-jin, actually fell in love, got married, and had a baby. What relief we all felt—reality trumped fiction!

"Together" Trumps "Divided"

The formation of the squad and its efforts against the evils that surround them are remarkable. I return to Audrey Jenkins's analysis of "care," mentioned in Chapter 1. She defined *jeong* as "a social phenomenon of warm, communal closeness, interdependency, and obligation to those with whom jeong is shared."[22] Jenkins arrived at the important conclusion that partition was a tool of anti-care, but *jeong* trumped partition and enabled good people on both sides to triumph over evil.

The word Jenkins chose—*jeong*—may not be exactly the right word. I think the bonds of *jeong* are more like what we in the US would call "strong" ties, the bonds of family, religion, hometown, and the "old school." My Korean teacher, Professor Park, suggested that 전우애 (*cheo-nu-eh*), the bonding of people who have fought together, might be more appropriate. It describes the bonding that goes on during empowered collaboration and that can make a powerful difference in one's life. Whatever word is used, Jenkins's point, that interpersonal concern and connection trump the anti-care of partition, is a profound one.

One great statement of care was that articulated by the African American diplomat Ralph Bunche in his lecture upon receiving the 1950 Nobel Peace Prize, in which he discussed his work with the newly formed United Nations. The lecture, given on December 11, 1950, took place as the Korean War was going on. Bunche articulated the arguments for the UN intervention in the Korean War, which were completely incompatible with the atrocities that followed. However, he set this fundamental standard for achieving peace:

> Peace, to have meaning for many who have known only suffering in both peace and war, must be translated into bread or rice, shelter, health, and education, as well as freedom and human dignity—a steadily better life. If peace is to be secure, long-suffering and long-starved, forgotten peoples of the world, the underprivileged and the undernourished, must begin to realize without delay the promise of a new day and a new life.[23]

Korea was wrenched willy-nilly into modernism by colonialism, the Korean War, and the rush to capitalism, none of which solved the issues Bunche raised. And the habits of the feudal past, which had lasted for such a long time, haunt both Koreas. All of K-drama reflects the jarring contrasts that endure. Some stories dive into points of the conflict, and *Crash Landing on You* is the great exemplar of this.

In a democracy we have a freewheeling system of recording history, and people with different points of view defiantly declare that their version is the right one. Within Korea, there is not much divergence in the ways the history of Japanese occupation is presented, at least that I've seen. But that consensus ends when World War II ends and the country is divided into two parts, with Americans in control of the south and Communists under the leadership of Kim Il Sung in control of the north. Some of the differences I've encountered have to do summaries of the facts. When I visited the DMZ, guides and exhibits argued that the UN forces "saved our country for us"—I've also heard this summarized as "saving the country for freedom and democracy." This is, at the very least, misleading, because South Korea was under a dictatorship for decades—there was no freedom or democracy. And how would the country have been "lost" if it had been unified by North Korea? It is not the country that would have been lost but rather the form of political economy, which is not at all the same thing.

The other problem in writing history lies in the choice of which facts to use. For example, at the War Memorial of Korea, the story of the Korean War centers around the invasion from the North and the pushback by the South. That jibes with what little I knew about Korean history before I became fascinated by K-drama. Yet other reports document that the UN forces did terrible damage in the north, basically destroying every village and town, forcing people to live in underground caves. The slogan at the War Memorial of Korea—"If you want peace, prepare for war"—captures an analysis of past events, which commits both sides to militarization and alliances with powerful nations who can fight alongside them.

But from my reading I learned of the vast destruction of the north and its rebuilding via Socialist solidarity, with many kinds of support from the Soviet Union, East Germany, and other countries of the Communist bloc. This history was new to me, and I'd say it is a history of *jeong*. It may help us understand North Korea's willingness in 2024 to send men and materiel to aid Russia in its war in Ukraine.

Into these conflicting narratives comes *Crash Landing on You*, which takes us "into the North" and provides a very sympathetic portrayal of life on the other side of the DMZ. One of the radical aspects of this show is that it takes us into the DMZ itself. This is a very large no man's land. That we watch people walking around in it—including our heroes Captain Ri and Yoon Se-ri—opens doors mentally. Like others I'm sure, I'm fascinated by the rewilding of the DMZ and would love to see it. Could peace be made and the mines removed so that we could go there and reconnect the two sides? We were able to go to the wild place of the High Line, a former elevated rail line in New York City, so why not the DMZ?

But it is not a trivial thing to ask to go to the DMZ. I worked with Dr. Véronique Héon-Klin on her study of the rise and fall of the Berlin Wall.[24] Though the differences between East and West Germany were not as great as those between North and South Korea, and the separation was shorter and less absolute, German reunification has been slow, difficult, and more costly than people imagined. That doesn't mean it shouldn't happen; rather, it means that it will take determination for it to happen. Like the 10 plagues that preceded the Exodus from Egypt, Korean reunification will take *something* that solidifies the people's wish for unity. And it will be followed by the proverbial 40 years in the wilderness as people resolve their profound differences.

While the wish for unity may fall short of the power needed to create reunification, the suffering resulting from division is

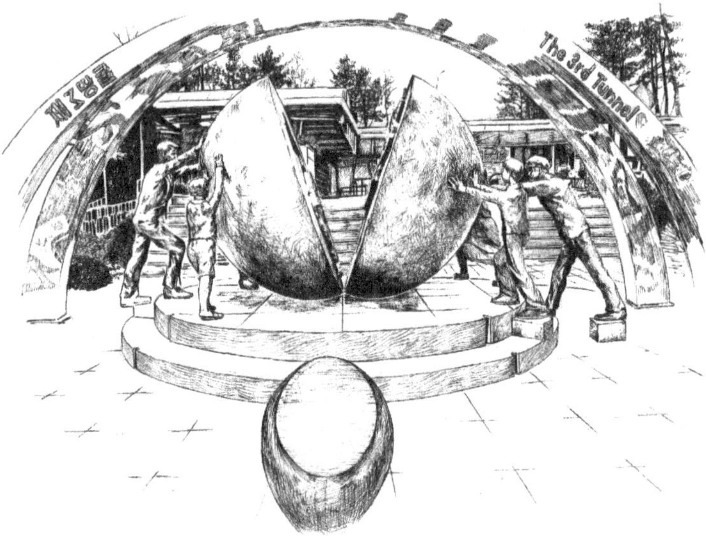

Figure 8.3 Split-Apart Halves.
This statue is in the demilitarized zone, at the site of the Third Invasion Tunnel.
Drawing by Mike Malbrough, used with permission.

enormous. Plato proposed the idea of the "split-apart half": the soul is split into two, and one half is placed in one person and the other half in another person. These two halves then search for each other so that they can be whole—Plato is much more complicated than that, but that's the gist of the popular version. In the DMZ, at the site of the Third Invasion Tunnel, there's a statue of a sphere cut in half. On the cut surfaces are maps, each with a raised and lowered piece. On one side, North Korea is raised but South Korea is lowered. On the other half, the opposite is the case. Then on the outside of the sphere there are people pushing the halves back together, to complete the map (Figure 8.3).

In *Crash Landing on You*, the wealthy heiress Yoon Se-ri represents South Korea, while the army captain Ri Jeong-hyeok represents North Korea, roles surely not chosen by accident. They fall in love as they are stripped of their roles. They desperately want to be together. At one point, after Yoon Se-ri was kidnapped by Ri Jeong-hyeok's powerful father, Captain Ri says to him, "I can't breathe without her." In my view, this stands for the longing of the split-apart halves of Korea to be rejoined, a profound dilemma that hangs over all of K-drama, over all of Korea, north and south. The unification is hindered by the factors that separated our lovers: wealth and might. Should South Korea share its wealth with the poorer North Korea? Should North Korea share its military might with South Korea? One message of *Crash Landing on You* is that true happiness does not lie in either of those directions; rather, it lies in human relationships. As Audrey Jenkins found, *jeong* is the source of happiness, while partition is anti-*jeong*.

This highlights the deeper problem—and the crucial dilemma—which is that the division was created and is maintained not by Koreans, but by dueling superpowers that have used the peninsula in their proxy wars. The Koreans are not powerless in this situation, but they do not hold all the power. The Sword of Damocles hangs over their heads, and indeed over all our heads. Can we take steps toward peace? How about just one?

9

Peace Between the Universes

Lee Gon Is in Time

I believe that the United States is at the crossroads. And time has run out. We have no more time for war, or exploitation, or poisoning the earth. We must learn to live together now

—Ernest Thompson, from *Homeboy Came to Orange*

Wield it with deep thoughts, Pyeha, and make things right.

—Written on the Four Tiger Sword, *The King: Eternal Monarch*

There is no crime more onerous than greed,
No misfortune more devastating than avarice.
And no calamity that brings with it more grief than insatiability.
Thus, knowing when enough is enough
Is really satisfying.

—*The Tao*, No. 46

At the end of every episode of *The King: Eternal Monarch*, we see an animation of a clock with its hands running backward. Figure 9.1 shows three snippets. In the end, the hands of the clock form the word 더 (the) for the first part of the title, "The King."

The king, Lee Gon, is a warrior, meaning he evidences both a clarity of purpose and a sense of great burden. Pádraig Ó Tuama's

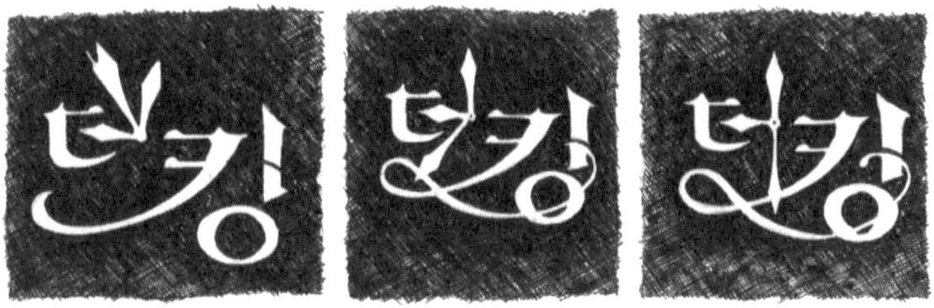

Figure 9.1 Losing Time.
An animation of hands on a clock running backward is shown at the end of each episode of *The King: Eternal Monarch.*
Drawing by Mike Malbrough, used with permission.

book *50 Poems to Open Your World* includes a poem called "A Blessing" by James Wright. Wright, a veteran who struggled in the aftermath of World War II, wrote about visiting two ponies in a field at twilight. "They bow shyly as wet swans. They love each other," observes Wright of their comradeship, to which he adds the melancholic qualification, "There is no loneliness like theirs." Ó Tuama notes, "It takes courage to welcome gladness while you're carrying something else."[1]

The "something else" in Lee Gon's case is that, at age 8, he witnessed the murder of his father by his uncle, who also tried to kill him. He was rescued by a mysterious masked stranger dressed all in black. He was left with a scar on his neck and two treasures—half of a magical flute and an ID card for "Jeong Tae-eul," a police lieutenant who does not exist in his country.

In the arc of restoration, the first phase is the yin of good/yang of evil, which pivots as grace touches the heart-mind. All of this happens in the first episode of *The King: Eternal Monarch*, but then Lee Gon is left in stasis. Blogger CollectsFallenStars explains that he lived by three rules:

- He doesn't eat food that hasn't been tasted beforehand.
- No one touches his body.
- No one can call him by his name.

Though in emotional stasis, he has grown into his role as king. It is Wonderland that opens the way for the parts to come together.

Going to Wonderland

Jeong Tae-eul's ID card is kept in Lee Gon's copy of *Alice in Wonderland.* The following excerpt explains how Alice got to Wonderland:

> There was nothing so very remarkable in that; nor did Alice think it so *very* much out of the way to hear the Rabbit say to itself, "Oh dear! Oh dear! I shall be late!" (when she thought it over afterwards, it occurred to her that she ought to have wondered at this, but at the time it all seemed quite natural); but when the Rabbit actually *took a watch out of its waistcoat-pocket* and looked at it, and then hurried on, Alice started to her feet, for it flashed across her mind that she had never before seen a rabbit with either a waistcoat-pocket, or a watch to take out of it, and burning with curiosity, she ran across the field after it, and fortunately was just in time to see it pop down a large rabbit-hole under the hedge.
>
> In another moment down went Alice after it, never once considering how in the world she was to get out again.[2]

Here is how Lee Gon got to Wonderland:

Dressed in his royal ceremonial hanbok, he takes *Alice in Wonderland* to read to children. Like Alice, who was bored sitting by her sister, the children are bored by his reading. They want to gossip about his love life. On learning he doesn't have a girlfriend, one prophetic child suggests he go down the rabbit hole and find one. And a few days later he does—jumping on Maximus, his white charger, to follow a person in a rabbit jacket. He loses track of that person but encounters a magical gate. He charges through and emerges in the Republic of Korea. There he meets Lieutenant Jeong Tae-eul, the woman he has been dreaming about since the day of the treason.

Such a preposterous set of circumstances! Fratricide, interdimensional travel, a gorgeous man without a girlfriend—we are flabbergasted at every turn and all that happened in the first hour. Let's pause a moment—it is essential to say that, in a world of gorgeous people, Lee Min-ho, who plays Lee Gon, rises to the next level. And that's part of what's so preposterous—how can people be so beautiful?

And! Such cool outfits! Jonathan Yeo's portrait of King Charles III, unveiled in 2024, has an eerie resemblance to Lee Gon's royal portrait in his sumptuous red robes. Surely Jonathan Yeo watches K-drama? Or maybe he studied the Korean art of royal portraits? The portraits also remind me of professor and painter Eunju Hwang's amazing zebra with a magenta mane, a painting she calls "I need a little color in my life!"

We all need a little color in our lives—these are hard times. The rabbit hole offers a way to the future, and that is why Lee Gon jumps into the unknown. Shortly after arriving in the Republic of Korea, he encounters Jeong Tae-eul. She warns him that it is against the law to ride his horse in Gwanghwamun, the historic center of Seoul. He pays no attention to her orders, distracted by his amazement that, after 25 years, she is actually in front of him. He hugs her, and she arrests him.

Faced with this person who says he is from another universe, Jeong Tae-eul, the police officer, seeks to manage a psychotic person. Lee Gon, on the other hand, rather calmly, keeps asserting his truth, the truth of his universe where he is king. When he asks for what he is entitled to have as a monarch, she puts him in a cell. When he asks for a chair, saying, "I've never sat on the floor," she ignores him. When she takes his watch and he requests she place it carefully on a pad, she drops it in a box. He restrains his anger. When he is released and needs money and a place to stay, she agrees to go to a jewelry shop with him so that he can sell one of his diamond buttons. Convinced that his "king act" will be exposed, she quips, "If he says it's a diamond, my name is Princess Diana."

When the jeweler then declares that he's never seen such a finely cut stone, Lee Gon suggests smugly that she tell the jeweler her name. Clearly, Korean boys can be just as annoying as American boys in that kind of situation.

Lee Gon has been committed to Jeong Tae-eul since age 8. When he finally meets her, his feelings must evolve. The person he imagined her to be is replaced by the reality of who she is. Now he must get to know the real Jeong Tae-eul. He is surprised by her brashness and swagger, both necessary to succeed in her job as a violent crimes detective. When he asks her how she became a police officer, he is captivated by her answer: "Not everyone can be brave, so I decided to become brave."

We see the shift in his behavior. When Jeong Tae-eul says his name, he looks at her with wonder. "I thought my name was not supposed to be spoken," he explains, "but I guess it was only supposed to be spoken by you."

He takes her hand in front of his colleagues in the Kingdom of Corea. They are shocked to see him touching someone else. He smiles at them, confirming that this is the woman he loves, has always loved.

Blogger Catches Fallen Stars argues that Lee Gon's consistent assertion of the truth, verified by the unfolding of events, is what makes it possible for him to win over Jeong Tae-eul. Having to win her over is good for him—the handsome King is the object of infinite feminine adoration in Corea. She is the key to both his heart and this other universe.

Meanwhile, when Jeong Tae-eul meets a man who says he is from a parallel universe, she has what in the US we call a "Show me" attitude, as in "I'm from Missouri, you have to show me." She is skeptical, to say the least, but she is also an able analyst, and as the data piles up, she shifts her stance. She is not entirely convinced until she arrives in his palace. In his magnificent study and surrounded by members of his court, the reality clicks. She is in the middle of speaking to him in informal speech—*banmal*—but corrects herself, replacing it with the deferential style of speech that indicates he is a person of high rank.

I was happy that Professor Park translated this segment for me, because the subtitles don't fully convey the subtlety of what is said:

Lee Gon: 상황 봐서 땡땡이 치고 올테니까. [After I assess what's going on, I'll play hooky and come back (said in *banmal*, the informal speech).]

Jeong Tae-eul: 보니까 매를 버네. [I noticed you're asking for it (she too uses *banmal*).]

She looks around and sees the horror on the faces of the people of his court. She rephrases: 매를 버십니다. [You're asking for it, sir (the "sir" conveys the change to honorific speech, but the same criticism is spoken to the king).]

She sees that people are still shocked and says softly to him: 이것도 아니구나. [This is not it either (using *banmal*).]

Lee Gon, speaking to his people, laughs and says: 이젠 진짜 믿어, 내가 황젠거. [Now she really trusts that I'm the king (he walks out chuckling).]

High court lady: 아이고 두야, 아이고 심이야 (also *banmal* but to herself). [*Aigoo* my head. *Aigoo* my heart. (word for "heart" derived from Chinese).]

Not only does Jeong Tae-eul respect the evidence, but also she is a woman who takes action. She is being courted by a charming and handsome man. When she is convinced he is the king, she does not hesitate to embrace her fate and say "I love you." She says this in Episode 8, way ahead of the usual confessions in Episode 10 or 11 of K-drama.

In time, the ebullience of the wooing will yield to time itself. Lee Gon becomes aware that time stops when the intergalactic gates are crossed and that as the number of crossings increases, time stops for longer and longer periods of time. He calculates that the periods of frozen time are increasing by the square of the prime number. Following a prime number table, he is able to predict that at the 63rd event, prime number 293, time will stop for a day, and then a month, and then for longer than we might be able to count.[3]

The traitorous uncle, Lee Lim, who possesses the other half of the magical flute, has used its powers to build a small army to promote his evil vision of infinite life and power. His use of power without counting the cost is what has profoundly disturbed the balance and threatens the existence of both worlds.

Program, Posse, and Paperclip

Lee Gon needs resources if he is to triumph. I think of these resources as "program, posse, and paperclip." The program is both the plan of action and the moral assumptions from which the plan emerges. The posse is the group of collaborators that will help him reach his goal. The paperclip refers to the MacGyver-like trick of making magic with what's at hand.[4]

Program

The term "program," as I use it, cements our moral values to the specific actions we will take to bring them into reality. Elucidating a program expresses our basic assumptions about how to live and work in the world.

From a young age, Lee Gon has been trained to lead the nation. The koan-like inscription on the Four Tiger Sword, a symbol of his status and his path, set a moral code:

> The sky bestows the heart upon us, and the ground helps the spirit.
> The sun and the moon are formed.
> As the mountains and streams form, lightning strikes.
> A sage is moved to defeat the evil of the mountains and streams.
> Wield it with deep thoughts, Pyeha, and make things right.

As a boy, when Lee Gon's father asks him if he will be able to adhere to that path, even if it means eating spinach and beans, he is hesitant. But at age 8, after seeing the corpse of his father, he does not hesitate to accept the role and its responsibilities: He tries to pick up the sword and avenge his father but succeeds only in cutting the magical flute, the *Manapasikjoek*, in half. His traitorous uncle flees the palace with one half—some power but all.

As an 8-year-old king, Lee Gon's first duty was to lead the funeral rites for the former king. In Korea, as it has been explained to me, funeral rites involve ceremonial wailing, which is not the same as crying. In the show, the boy wails for his father during the ceremony, whereas when he is alone with the high court lady, he weeps. In an unusual move, this show compresses the trauma and the moment of grace into the first episode. Key to that grace are the actions of the high court lady, who, among other acts, connects him with Jo Yeong; upon seeing Lee Gon's suffering, Jo Yeong commits himself to being his ally and "unbreakable sword."

Lee Gon grows up to be a poised and accomplished man. When he has gone down the rabbit hole and jumped universes, Lieutenant Jeong Tae-eul asks if someone taught him to say the gracious things that led everyone at the palace to adore him. Lee Gon explains that he taught himself. We can understand this as him having become a master of *nunchi*, the Korean skill of reading a room and working to make the interactions in it successful.[5] We can also understand it as a way to keep at a distance and maintain watchfulness.

The Posse

The formation of the posse reminds me of the old question "Do you want to be part of the problem or part of the solution?"

My father pushed through a terrible terminal illness so that he might finish his book, *Homeboy Came to Orange: A Story of People's Power*. He thought the key lesson was coalition—that to build people's power, different groups of people could unite around a common cause. What K-drama has taught me is that his book holds another lesson: that trauma and loss can be healed by friends and that friends can work together to make the world better.

At his lowest point—when his work had been decimated by the brutal attacks of McCarthyism—Dad met Dr. John Alexander, a young pediatrician who lived around the corner from us. In my dad's papers there is a fragment of a tribute he made to Dr. Alexander, in which he said that Doc became his friend when he needed a friend. That friendship led to other friendships, to the fight to desegregate the Orange, New Jersey, public schools, and to years of organizing for people's power. As others connected to the struggle, the friendship between Dad and Doc enlarged to include Ben Jones, Molly Brown, Rudy Thomas, Preston Grimsley, Becky Doggett, Ed Andrade, and many others. The circle of friends changed the city and changed themselves. That is the story of a posse.

The formation of the posse is fundamental to the process of restoration that K-drama is teaching us. We can think of the two universes—the Kingdom of Corea and the Republic of Korea—as an ellipsis, with two centers, one revolving around King Lee Gon and the other revolving around Lieutenant Jeong Tae-eul. But that analogy leaves out the interdimensional space, the road of thunder and lightning that connects the two. The parallel to the demilitarized zone is clear for all to see. Compare this diagram shown in Figure 9.2 to the map of Korea in Chapter 8 (Figure 8.1).

Despite his clear values and social skills, Lee Gon faces the complicated challenge of pulling together a posse across two universes. In his home universe, he has long-standing relationships and can draw on his vast wealth and the goodwill he has built. We see how he cultivates this goodwill when at one point he asks the team working in the kingdom's data center to find Jeong Tae-eul: "I am not ordering," he explains. "I'm asking."

> After he has saved her, Jeong Tae-eul asks, "How did you find me?" Lee Gon replies, "I told you I'm a decent person in this Universe."
>
> In Jeong Tae-eul's universe, Lee Gon knows no one. There he starts off with nothing more than the diamond buttons on his

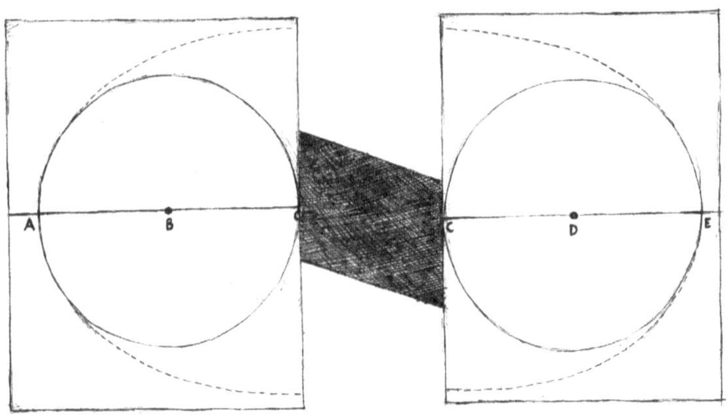

Figure 9.2 The Ellipsis.
The two worlds of the show are connected by a "road of thunder and lightning."
Drawing by Mike Malbrough, used with permission.

> jacket. So how does he make friends and win allies there? We see him first make friends with Jo Eun-sup, Jeong Tae-eul's dear friend. They go shopping and arrive back at Lee Gon's hotel with bags and bags of clothes. Lee Gon says to Jo Eun-sup, "What's in your left hand is for me; what's in your right hand is for you." Winning over coffee shop owner Myeong Na-ri and Jeong Tae-eul's dad is also easy—both take Lee Gon at face value, and respectful exchanges lead to friendship.
>
> Kang Sin-jae, by contrast, is the rival suitor and antagonistic to Lee Gon. He is also someone who was brought over from the kingdom to the republic, though he has amnesia about that shift. As his memories come into focus, he shifts much—but not all—of that anger to Lee Lim. Kang Sin-jae is sensitive to moral ambiguity and deceit, but Lee Gon has none of that: this is what will win over Kang Sin-jae to Lee Gon's side.

Joined across the universes, this complex group of people forms an empowered collaboration, a term I invented to describe ad hoc groups that assemble to manage a situation and empower themselves with knowledge and a system of decision-making.[6]

The Paperclip

MacGyver does magic with paperclips, but Lee Gon has an actual magical artifact: the *Manapasikjoek*, a magical flute that had been given to his ancestor. The full powers of the flute are never explained, but we do know that it can open portals to other worlds. That is how Lee Gon can move from the Kingdom of Corea to the Republic of Korea. Because the flute was cut in half, his murderous uncle, Lee Lim, has half, and Lee Gon has half. We encounter again the trope of the split-apart halves destabilizing the world while apart and needing to be reunited.

Taking on Evil

With program, posse, and paperclips in hand, the show moves to the confrontation with evil.

> After killing his brother, the king, in 1994, Lee Lim ran from the scene into the bamboo forest carrying with him half of the *Manapasikjoek*, the magic flute, which he uses to open a portal. He had heard of this from his father, so the moment confirms that the power he was seeking is in his hands. He goes through the portal and finds himself in the Republic of Korea, where he immediately begins to kill people who are the doppelgangers of his family. He has powers—never fully explained—because of the flute. He uses these to build a shadow army, half in the Republic of Korea and half in the Kingdom of Corea. His evil has tendrils that reach out to entangle people he needs for their money or their talents, offering them untold riches and requiring that they kill their doppelganger, as he has, in order to become part of his empire.

Lee Lim builds his power based on appealing to people's greed, revenge, and hate and enforcing their commitment with violence should they stray. He is clearly a sadist who takes pleasure in hurting others. I am reminded that Chapter 53 of *The Tao* reminds us that highway robbery should not be confused with way-making.

Jack Nicholson, in the film *A Few Good Men*, alleges that society doesn't want to know what he, as a solider, has to do to protect our freedoms. This speech concludes with the famous line "You don't want the truth—you can't handle the truth." In general, I find that I shy away from the truth, and this K-drama reminded me that I steer toward the cheerful, if possible. It was on the 67th viewing of the show—I exaggerate slightly—that I began to grapple with Lee Gon's use of violence. There is a crucial set of scenes that inform us that he is not a warrior in theory, but someone trained at the Naval Academy, 88th class, and the commander in chief of the country's forces. He joins a battleship during a confrontation with Japan and forces their vessels to retreat from Corea's waters.

When he learns about the hideout of some of Lee Lim's followers, Lee Gon takes his guard there. The leader of the guard asks what he wants to happen in the surprise attack, and he replies, "Kill them." Twenty to 30 traitors are shot dead on the spot. Later, Lee Lim kidnaps Jeong Tae-eul, and Lee Gon throws his guard, the police, and other forces at Lee Lim's men. Another 20 or 30 people are killed. When Lee Gon orders the beheading of a traitor, the traitor protests that beheading was eliminated in the 1920s. Lee Gon replies, "You've been away from the kingdom for a while and you've forgotten that my word is law."

As an American raised on gratuitous violence, I am satisfied by these scenes—they seem necessary in the context of the struggle and different from Lee Lim's sadism. But having acknowledged these acts as violence, I started to think about things like due process and having a private army that can kill. December is the time of Christmas carols, and a friend pointed out that the song "I Heard the Bells on Christmas Day" is from a Civil War–era poem by Henry Wadsworth Longfellow. This song is a favorite of my granddaughter Lily and juxtaposes the despair of war with the hope of peace. What is necessary and right to defeat evil?

Because this is the "Tao of K-drama," it is useful to return to *The Tao*'s admonition not to use coercion. In my view, *The Tao* was written as advice for leaders—it was written for Lee Gon. *The Tao* does not forbid violence; it forbids coercion. Lee Lim uses coercion all the time. Lee Gon counters aggression with force, but he does not coerce people. When he is frantic to find Jeong Tae-eul, he asks politely for the data center to help him. A coercion-versus-noncoercion debate is different, I think, from that about violence versus nonviolence, and each throws light on the other.

Who Will Help Me Plant the Wheat? I Will! I Will! I Will! I Will!

In the children's story about the Little Red Hen, the other animals don't want to do the work—they just want to eat the bread. The posse that joins around Lee Gon is quite the opposite. Each one wants to shoulder the burden to accomplish the goal and, if possible, to spare Lee Gon. While Lee Gon did much to win loyalty and admiration, it is also because he has changed, making deeper and more open connections with people. As he welcomed people into his world, they became committed to battle with and for him and against Lee Lim.

With time literally running out, Lee Gon must move into action. His first aborted attempt to go to the past to stop Lee Lim leads him to reconsider his plan. He decides that he must go back in time again, this time to sacrifice himself. As a king this would certainly seem to be in the purview of his powers and duties. But to pull this off, he needs the support of the posse he has gathered. At one point Lee Gon says, "I hoped that everything would unfold as it did last time."

The posse, each wanting to do their part, was not willing to stay on the sidelines as the confrontation with evil moved to its denouement. Lee Gon realizes that the posse has come to the showdown with him. "What is different this time?" he asks and concludes, "I am not alone."

This decision is very typical of his abilities as a leader. He had set out, in a traditional hero manner, to shoulder the burden himself. When he realizes that is not what is going to happen, he adapts.

When the final confrontation occurs, Lee Gon recites the whole verse from the sword, emphasizing, "Wield it with deep thoughts, Pyeha, and set things right." He condemns the traitor

> to be beheaded and carries out the sentence without a moment's hesitation. He has held that moment in his mind for a long time, and he performs it with conviction.

With the death of the traitor on the night of the treason in 1994, time resets. In the intermediate zone we see a watch spin wildly—time rewinding. I made the point in Chapter 2 that having a party at the end of a long process is one of the SmallGestures that promote change. Many shows end with a party, but *The King: Eternal Monarch* is an exception. Because the king had to go back into the past to change the outcome, his posse then lived in a future in which none of their collective work happened. Only Lee Gon, Jeong Tae-eul, and Jo Yeong remember. There is sorrow in that, but all three understand that it was their fate to bear this sorrow and to live in the only possible future they could make. That is, in its own way, I think, a profound celebration.

Empowered Collaboration and Putting Patterns on the World

Robert Coles, who studied African American children involved in the civil rights movement of the 1960s, noted:

> It must be said that under great stress [the children] have somehow done more than persist, more than endure. They have prevailed ... by summoning every bit of their humanity in the face of every effort made to deny any of it to them. In so doing, they have become more than they were, more than they themselves thought they were, and perhaps more than anyone watching them can't quite put to word: bearers and makers of tradition; children who in the moment—call it existential, call it historical, call it psychological—took what they had from the past, in their

minds, out of their homes, and made of *all* those possessions something else: a change in the world, and in themselves.[7]

Lee Gon has been changed in that way. For years, he held himself at a distance from the world, not able to be touched or to be called by name. He went down the rabbit hole out of a great need to resolve the tragedy that lay on his heart and in his life. The empowered collaboration across two universes enabled him to leave those restrictions behind, to test himself against the threat to the world, and to emerge able to love fully and freely. With his interdimensional posse, he made a change in the worlds and in himself.

Just as Robert Coles was astounded by what happened to the children of crisis, so too am I astounded by the transformation of Lee Gon. It is not accomplished by psychotherapy; it is not small; it is not slow. It happened by engagement with others in the struggle against massive evil. This is what the great philosophers were telling us about the complexity and adaptability of people, and about their power to put new patterns on the world. May it hearten us to know that we can find ways to stop evil and return the balance to our world.

10

Tides of Hope

Keep us forever on the path, we pray.

—*Lift Every Voice and Sing*, James Weldon Johnson

Dr. Kim Sabu always tells us, "Don't stop asking yourself why we are living and what we're living for. The moment we give up on that question will be the end of our romance in life. All right?" And that's what he tells us.

—Dr. Seo Woo-jin, in *Dr. Romantic*

Do not reduce the size of [the common people's] residence
And do not lower their standard of living.
It is only because you do not lower their standard of living
That they do not become disaffected.

—*The Tao*, No. 72

The *Tao Te Ching* gives us a set of parameters for living a life of significance. These concepts are part of the deep heritage of Korea, and they are infused in K-drama as the narrative arc of restoration. The Tao of K-drama teaches us that the injured self can be healed, can rejoin the collective, and then can help to make a change in the world. The Tao of K-drama emphasizes that we are not healing the self solely for the self but to become *oori* (Korean for "we the family of us") so that we are all riding the waves—searching for the keys to be a collective, held together by love, in spite of precarity and buoyed by joy. The goal of situation analysis is to "name the situation." *Tides of Hope* was the title my 2024 situation analysis class settled on after studying *Our Blues,* and this is a way of articulating what the narratives of K-drama are instilling in us.

K-drama, by offering us the narrative arc of restoration, gives us a model of the world that is big enough and other-centered enough for us to face our massive troubles while staying hopeful. This is a major cognitive shift from the "happy ending" narrative. As Yoon Ji-ho says in *Because This Is My First Life*, shows end with the kiss because what comes after the kiss is reality, which can be very painful or very dark.[3] The "happily ever after" narratives that stop at the kiss or the marriage teach us to focus on the magical moment of finding love. They give us no tools for facing the aftermath—reality—and so it is a very small narrative frame. The narrative arc of restoration uses the kiss as the springboard to traverse the hard parts while teaching us to join with others so that we can face these hard parts as a posse rather than alone. It is a very large frame, large enough for the problems of our troubled world.

Narrative frames are fundamental to how we think, and cognitive therapies have been developed that help us recognize the frame from which we are working and shift it to something more serviceable. These are so intuitive that Eleanor Porter wrote about cognitive therapy for depression and Bill Wilson explained the shift from the logic of alcoholism to the logic of sobriety long before Dr. Aaron Beck's research established cognitive behavioral therapy.[4] And K-dramas are so delightful that we are reminded that a little bit of sugar helps the medicine go down!

My Story of Encountering the Tao of K-Drama

Alone with my Netflix button in the middle of the COVID-19 pandemic, I encountered a story about a complete jerk who became enlightened and a much better person. How? I asked, stunned that the show cared, and even more stunned that the change had happened. I went down the rabbit hole in search of understanding. Like Alice, or like Lee Gon, I found myself in a new world—with a new language, new ideas, new storylines, and new endings. I was charmed and fascinated from the beginning.

I leaned in.

Perhaps it's obvious in retrospect that what I really wanted was to be enlightened, the way Heo Im was, via kindness, welcome, and the occasional rap on the knuckles. I didn't think that watching TV would change me; however, people working in narrative medicine have observed the powerful role that stories can play in our lives. I was alone, these were my new friends, one thing led to another, and my being shifted.

Part of the way this unfolded was that I announced to everyone that I was going to go to Korea for three months. I'm not someone who likes adventures. In fact, when friends would say, "You're going to have an adventure," I would reply, "No, I'm simply going to go to Korea and find a nice coffee shop." That is, I said that until three weeks before I was to leave, when total panic hit me: I was going to Korea for three months by myself! At this point, my tune changed. I begged Professor Park to show me on a map where I was going and how I might find food. Looking back, this actually was the funniest part of my terror, because the easiest thing to find in Seoul is food! Really, really good food.

At the time I didn't think of K-drama as a White Rabbit. I didn't think I was Heo Im or Lee Gon, changing my life by taking a chance. Just around the corner from my lodging in Itaewon was a restaurant named Dear Alice, which had a lovely neon rabbit displayed outside. I swear that rabbit winked at me every time I passed (Figure 10.1).

I was met with incredible kindness in Korea but also experienced enough of the hard edges to know I wasn't in a fantasy. I went on a temple stay and slept on the hard floor and was visited by some beetles, which had no fear because they'd evolved for hundreds of

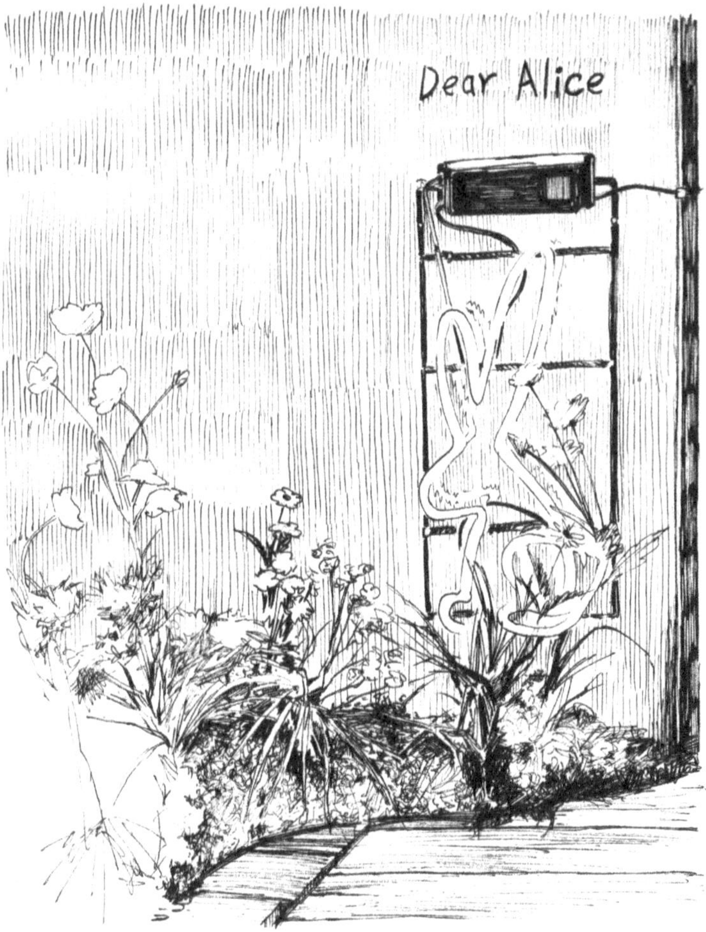

Figure 10.1 The Rabbit Who Winked
This neon sign is placed at the entrance to the Itaewon restaurant, Dear Alice.

years in a place where they were not hurt by people. I went to a doctor who took care of every aspect of my being. I went to a language school that didn't care that I was old and slow, and another that worked at my pace. I went to the War Museum and saw boys in uniform who, like me, were reading that the way to peace was to prepare for war. I took so many buses and got lost so many times. I met a psychiatrist who paid such close attention to what I said and how I said it that I almost fell out of my chair. And I made a friend who got me the best possible care when I had COVID and another who sent me wonderful bread and coffee so that I could get well. Friends and family came and went during my adventure, last of whom was Jae Shin, who took my 나무 친구 (Tree Friend) to Professor Hwang, who took it to live in Byun Jeong Dae-seob's beautiful garden.

It was all Grace offered to me, and, like Heo Im, I shifted. I think that is how the light gets in—it's not the crack, as Leonard Cohen proposed, because the crack hurts. It's Grace, which soothes and heartens us and allows us to open to the light. Some would say this is semantics, but watch K-drama and you'll see I'm right about the order.

In any event, the shift in my thinking became apparent during a June 2024 trip to Worchester, Massachusetts. I had driven there to give grand rounds to the Department of Psychiatry at the University of Massachusetts Chan School of Medicine. On arrival, I drove past the city's old industrial sector to its periphery with its new mall-style developments. To get to my hotel, I drove onto park-like grounds, past a solid, Victorian building. I sensed (in my bones, you might say) that I was on the grounds of an old mental hospital. I went for a walk on the grounds and that sense rapidly developed into a profound feeling of homecoming—I had trained in psychiatry in a hospital of similar vintage located in park-like grounds. I explored further and found where the old psychiatric hospital had stood, close to which the new hospital was located. A clock tower, salvaged from the old hospital, had been reconstructed on a stone terrace, where it stood like a guiding light. At one end of the terrace I encountered, carved in the granite, these words by the Scottish writer and social reformer Samuel Smiles: "Hope is like the sun, which, as we journey towards it, casts the shadow of our burden behind us."

"Hope is like the sun" quickly became "Hope like the sun!," which has been my mantra ever since.

Before watching K-drama, I would say to people that I didn't believe in "hope," as it is usually about specifying an outcome, which is too limited a way to look at the world. But I found that I resonated deeply with Samuel Smiles's affirmation, and I was so surprised! In the course of my efforts to understand K-drama, I had changed, but how? One way to describe this cognitive shift was that I understood a new, transcendental Hope, with a capital "H." Vaclav Havel, former president of the Czech Republic, spoke of this kind of Hope as "an orientation of the spirit, an orientation of the heart."[5]

Havel went on to say:

> It transcends the world that is immediately experienced, and is anchored somewhere beyond its horizons. . . . I feel that its deepest roots are in the transcendental, just as the roots of human responsibility are, though of course I can't—unlike Christians, for instance—say anything about the transcendental. . . .
>
> Hope, in this deep and powerful sense, is not the same as joy that things are going well, or willingness to invest in enterprises that are obviously headed for early success, but rather an ability to work for something because it is good, not just because it stands a chance to succeed. The more unpromising the situation in which we demonstrate hope, the deeper that hope is. Hope is not the same thing as optimism. It is not the conviction that something will turn out well, but the certainty that something makes sense, regardless of how it turns out. In short, I think that the deepest and most important form of hope, the only one that can keep us above water and urge us to good works, and the only true source

> of the breathtaking dimension of the human spirit and its efforts, is something we get, as it were, from "elsewhere." It is also this hope, above all, that gives us the strength to live and continually to try new things, even in conditions that seem as hopeless as ours do, here and now.[6]

Reverend Dr. Cynthia Bourgeault called this "mystical hope," a force that flows from the universe.[7] As Reverend Dr. Grace Ji-Sun Kim would say, it is Spirit in all its names, including Chi.[8] K-drama has many ways to teach us about this, but the most powerful is that it shows us the arc of restoration, which is itself like a wave, and the tides of Hope like the Sun.

Into Action

Every once in a while, we get to try out what we are learning. In the spring semester of 2024, my last semester teaching at The New School, I agreed to teach a class of undergraduates. I presumed this would be challenging. The undergraduates in my fall 2023 course, Political Economy of the City, had had a lot of trouble finishing the work and two had walked away, accepting a failing grade. I was shocked and disturbed—I had never had that happen before. I knew I needed a careful approach if my spring class were to be a success.

Because it was the 20th anniversary of the publication of my book *Root Shock*, there were a series of anniversary events going on, and I wanted to integrate the class into that process. I didn't anticipate the large number of students—18!—who showed up, which increased my fears. What I proposed to the class was that we read the book and make an exhibit to be shown somewhere.

I was intimidated, to say the least. And my fears seemed confirmed when the students showed up to the second class having barely skimmed the first chapter of the book, not bothering to look up words or references they didn't understand. I knew we were headed for disaster. I had a Great Power moment and yelled at them. I said, "You all are smart enough to be at Harvard where you'd be reading two books a week. We're reading one chapter a week, so don't show up without understanding every word."

They looked at me so blankly that I realized they had no idea what I wanted them to do. I told them to open their books to page 101, which contained excerpts from an interview with Mr. Charles Meadows, an older man who had lived through urban renewal in Roanoke, Virginia.

He opens by saying:

> Well it—all—winds down to a very small note.
> It seemed to me—, through the years,
> and I've been here a good little while,
> that when the black community got together,
> or they were segregated,
> they had to stay in one corner of the city.
> There were boundary lines everywhere.
> And—for some reason or another they stayed more healthier.
> They—were more protective to the families in the neighborhood
> and whatnot.[9]

After reading that small segment, we started to talk about it. We discussed the way I had chosen to format the excerpt, the way in which Mr. Meadows talked, and the content of what he was saying—the surprising assertion that the Black community was healthier during segregation.

It turns out that the students had a lot to say and every phrase was worth investigating. It opened up their curiosity and invited them to be inventive. Just as curiosity about Ha Mun-su was what got Lee Gang-du moving out of being stuck, so too did curiosity get my class moving. They shared with me that they had not read in that manner before—it was new and they enjoyed it. They became curious.

From some of their comments, I realized that they all thought that displacement—root shock—was something that happened to other people. So I said, "You know, you all have been through root shock."

They looked at me skeptically. I continued, "You were in high school at the time of the COVID shelter in place. That was root shock. What happened to you?"

To investigate this, I asked them to break up into pairs and interview each other. The stories turned out to be astounding. One of the most remarkable was the story of a French horn player who was going to play with her orchestra at Disney World but could not. The shared displacement was the Grace that touched us all.

At the next class a number of people were missing. I am not a patient person, and absence is rather intolerable to me. But I knew that I had failed my traumatized undergraduates in the fall semester and I needed a new approach. So I took on the problem of absences indirectly and asked those who were present, "What is hard about teamwork?"

The students had an immediate gut reaction: not everyone pulls their weight, people don't communicate or they wait days to respond to a text, some people take over the project, some want all the credit, *some don't show up*. It was a substantial list.

Then I asked, "So why do teamwork?"

Their answers were equally emphatic. One answered, "Because the work is better."

Another added, "You have more ideas, so the result is stronger."

A third agreed and said, "You can't do it alone."

I was struck by the consensus that teamwork, though hard, was simply better. We opened the door to becoming a posse.

Somewhere along the way, I remembered that my colleague Bill Morrish always gave students things like little notebooks he got at Muji, the fancy Japanese store that has a branch near The New School. So I got little notebooks and pencils for my students. Then I thought, what else could I give them? Valentine's candy, of course—I asked them all to be my Valentine. What else? When we finally planned to show the exhibit in the Orange Public Library and were going there to visit, I gave them each money for a train ticket *and* a snack. The more I focused on their well-being, the more the quality of their work went up. SmallGestures, all.

I knew that we had to work on the exhibit and that I had to make this as active and clear as possible. Both of these approaches are part of being "trauma informed." This also allowed them to see and enjoy one another's contributions and to feel increasingly secure in the group. By the time the end of the semester arrived, we were a coherent and joyful lot. Our group photo was taken at our last class, held at an outdoor restaurant (Figure 10.2).

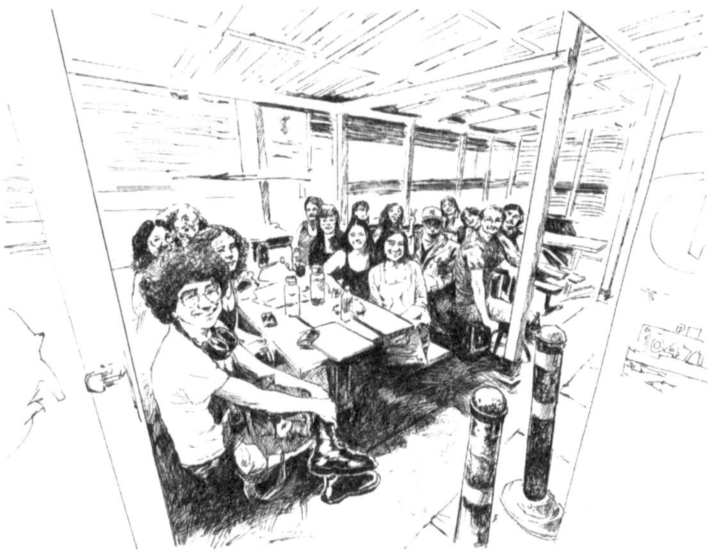

Figure 10.2 Our Class Celebrates.
My class and I gathered at an outdoor space on Sixth Avenue to celebrate our accomplishment.
Drawing by Mike Malbrough, used with permission.

We installed a lovely exhibit in the Stickler Memorial Library, the public library in Orange, New Jersey. We put the students' ingenuity and brave ideas on display in a city threatened by the root shock of gentrification. Their statement in that space has ripples: the posse made a change in the world.

Course evaluations are a very imprecise measure of what happens in a course—the people who fill them out typically really liked it or really didn't. But the comments made by the six students who did complete the evaluation confirmed that being trauma informed and building the collective had led to a positive experience.

One wrote, "Mindy is an incredible Professor who created a nurturing space for students to learn about the severity of Root Shock and urban renewal. Because of her teachings, I was introduced to new worlds and stories that will stay with me for the remainder of my lifetime."

Another, in Joycean free flow—maybe Mr. Meadows's style—wrote, "Having each student lead the readings helped us hear everyone's interpretations of the materials in new and creative ways the socratic discussion elements that discouraged everyone jumping into the most confident voice's plan in depth reading of one book allowed us to do some actual deep reading/reflection/analysis there was an opportunity for each student to bring their strength/talent into the class project although we were reading Root Shock, I felt like the purpose of this class was to teach us how to learn collaboratively."

Add your own punctuation to that one!

Figure 10.3 shows photographs of the exhibit they created. It was installed in the Orange Public Library, in two alcoves. The alcoves had housed a previous exhibit created by the University of Orange as part of a "reverse archeology" of the highway that had bisected the city in the 1960s. The students repurposed the existing six shadow boxes to hold storyboards they had created on the six topics they had chosen.

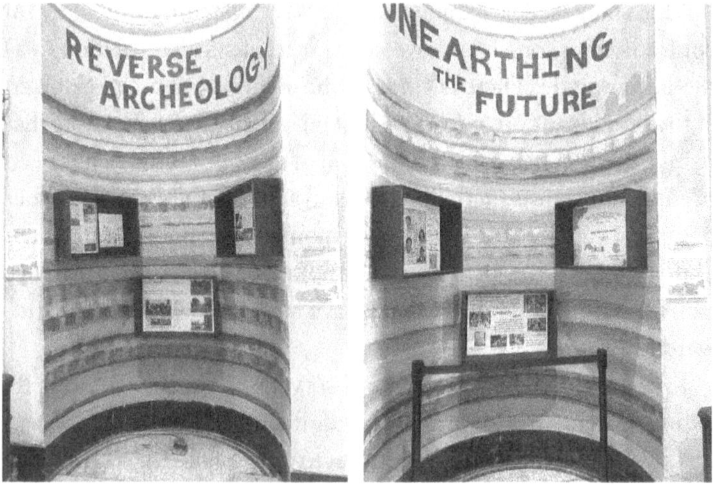

Figure 10.3 The Exhibit.
The class exhibit was installed at the Orange Public Library, May 24, 2024.
Installation originally created by Mike Malbrough. Photographs by Chloe Rousch, used with permission.

About the Narratives of K-Drama

K-dramas did not teach me to have hope because everything works out in the end, as occurs in American rom-coms. Rather, K-dramas accomplished this task because they showed me how people try—to recover, to work together, to be good.[10] They show us the way in which Chi shifts from being stuck to moving again. They show us the possibility of Grace that is given and received.

In a K-drama, Grace is always placed in the context of the stunning weight of the past and the challenges of the present. Precarity, avarice, profound destruction, and slim chances are always present in the stories. We can believe the stories because things are HARD. But, perhaps because change is the only constant, we are also shown that one can be quite Zen about everything, with a deep inner calm that makes it easier to take the moral position, to go out on a limb, to be in danger.

That may seem paradoxical, but by watching the flow of contradictions, one can move at a time that seems propitious—as the Bard noted, "There is a tide in the affairs of men, which taken at the flood leads on to fortune."[11] And one can move in a way that helps the collective, which is the goal of *nunchi*. This idea has been useful to me. Life is incredibly stressful at times, but I can be calmer because I can see that the present moment is one in a long chain that stretches from behind and continues in front of us. My eye cannot discern the full arc, but I have faith that we can bend it toward justice.

K-drama offers a vast set of observations on this subject. By telling so many stories, in so many domains, and with such varied casts of characters, K-drama helps us to understand the happenings at these various levels of scale. Even in the seven shows I have discussed here, we see a story about peace among the universes (*The King: Eternal Monarch*), peace between nations (*Crash Landing on You*), peace in the nation (*The King's Affection*), peace in the cities (*Just between Lovers*), peace among neighbors (*Prison Playbook*), peace in the home (*Romance Is a Bonus Book*), and peace in the heart (*Live Up to Your Name*). Giving us food for our imaginations is one of the roles of stories. We might complain that K-drama is not "realistic," but of course that is the point of fables—by giving us the gift of the fabulous, K-drama allows us to finally see the program, the posse, and the paperclips needed to put new patterns on the world.

Furthermore, we can see that the genre, as a whole, can be taken as a single soap opera. When I first started studying K-drama, I thought it was quite different from the US soap operas like *General Hospital*. But there are powerful strands among the many stories: a set of actors who reappear, scenes of the major cities and rural areas we get to know, tropes that require multiple investigations, and the deep sense of "We Are Korea" that pervades each individual story and links it to the larger whole: Jun Bum Sun's "emergence of a Korean archetype." Understanding that no story exists in isolation and no story simply has a happy ending helps me find my footing in difficult times. I can open my eyes, look around, and perceive the complexity of community all around me. I can replace the fallacious "Hero's Tale" with the "Story of Us," the web of life in which we all find ourselves. At last, I can fully appreciate Bill Morrish's diagram of the web of stories (see Figure 2.7).

When we watch K-dramas, we are watching fables about being a good person and having a significant life. They are not true stories. But they are not *not* true stories: they are stories of things that real people really do—get lost, find themselves confused, encounter a friend, define a purpose, and act to make the world better.

We too do these things.

And what a relief to know all this, because if ever there was a time when we need to act in concert, guided by deep moral values, it is now. I have learned from K-drama that we can have Hope.

And Therefore, We Hope Like the Sun!

I get *The New York Times* delivered to my home. I had COVID my last week in Korea, and I was pretty out of it when I first landed in New York. It wasn't until I'd been home for a few days that I noticed the front page of the newspaper, which portrayed a heart-wrenching photo of teenagers in one of the cities in Ukraine that had been devastated by war. The next day we had a lot of rain and my paper was wet, which amplified the impact of the terrible front-page photo of a young girl in Jakarta walking though the rising water that is filling her city. As I had eaten a lot of rice in Korea—Professor Park had taught me that the way to greet someone there is to ask, "Have you eaten rice today?"—the next day's front-page photo of the threat to the rice farms in Vietnam really hit home.

What does K-drama have to say to all of that?

Korea has been invaded as many as 800 times.[12] They know what root shock is—the pain of upheaval that never quite goes away but rather leaves behind a residue of *han* as both an ache and rage over what has been lost and an inspiration to hold tight to home and country. Korea is currently held apart by the terrible forces of global imperialism. K-drama, with all its intimacy and hit songs, shares with us a scrapbook of stories to say, "This is the Way we tackle our inheritance of pain and love."

I think K-drama is popular around the world because half a billion people have heard the message and taken heart.[13]

One of the roots of social psychiatry was in the effort of psychiatrists to lift the morale of the airmen in World War II who were going to fly missions, many to their death. Clifford Hunter, my mother's first husband, was one of those who chose to go into the sky to fight the fascists and save our democracy. For psychiatrists, the secret lay in the devotion to the team. Cliff Hunter lost his life because, when his plane crashed in the English Channel, he went back into the water to save his crewmate.

The Tao of K-drama teaches us that my individual salvation is not the goal but rather that my abilities, once freed from the straightjacket of my history, can become a resource for the ensemble. Together we can make a change in the world. But not just any change—change that is in step with the Way. As we sing in the Negro National Anthem, *Lift Every Voice and Sing*, "Keep us forever on the path, we pray."

APPENDIX 1

The 88 Shows on Which the Book Is Based

This analysis is based on 88 shows, viewed between January 2021 and August 2025.

Table A.1 Shows on Which the Book Is Based

Name of Show	Year
100 Days My Prince	2018
Because This Is My First Life	2022
Behind Your Touch	2023
Black Dog: Being a Teacher	2019
Boys over Flowers	2009
Bride of Habaek	2017*
Business Proposal	2022†
Cafe Minamdang	2022
Captivating the King	2024
Chocolate	2019*
Cinderella and the Four Knights	2016*
Coffee Prince	2007
Crash Course in Romance	2023
Crash Landing on You	2019†
The Crowned Clown	2019
Deep Rooted Tree	2011
Destined with You	2023
DP 1	2021
DP 2	2023
Dr. Romantic 1	2016
Dr. Romantic 2	2020
Dr. Romantic 3	2023†
Doctor Slump	2024
Do Do Sol Sol La La Sol	2020
Extraordinary Attorney Woo	2022†
Flower Crew: Joseon Marriage Agency	2019
Forecasting Love and Weather	2022

Table A.1 *Continued*

Name of Show	Year
The Good Doctor	2013
The Good Detective	2020
Goblin (Guardian: The Lonely and Great God)	2016*
Gyeongseong Creature	2023
Her Private Life	2019
Hometown Cha-Cha-Cha	2021*
Hospital Playlist 1	2020*
Hospital Playlist 2	2021*
Hotel Del Luna	2019
The Inheritors (The Heirs)	2013
Itaewon Class	2020
It's Okay Not to Be Okay	2020
Joseon Attorney: A Morality	2023
Just Between Lovers (Rain or Shine)	2017*
King the Land	2023*
The King: Eternal Monarch	2020*†
The King's Affection	2021*
Live Up to Your Name	2017
Love Next Door	2024
Mad for Each Other	2021
Man to Man	2017
Melo Movie	2025
Misaeng: Incomplete Life	2014*
Mr. Plankton	2024
Mr. Queen	2020†
Mr. Sunshine	2018
My Demon	2023
My Liberation Notes	2022*
My Love from the Stars	2013
My Mister	2019
My Only Love Song	2017
Mystic Pop-up Bar	2020
Navillera	2016†
Once Upon a Small Town	2022†
One Spring Night	2019*
Our Blues	2022*
Poong, the Joseon Psychiatrist	2022
Poong, the Joseon Psychiatrist 2	2023
Prison Playbook	2017*†
Racket Boys	2021
Record of Youth	2020

Table A.1 *Continued*

Name of Show	Year
Romance Is a Bonus Book	2019
Rookie Historian Goo Hae-ryung	2019*
Run On	2020
She Would Never Know	2021
Secret Garden	2010
Secret Royal Inspector and Joy	2021
See You in My 19th Life	2023
Signal	2016
Something in the Rain	2018
Stranger 1	2017
Stranger 2	2020
Summer Strike	2022
Touch Your Heart	2019*
The Trauma Code: Heroes on Call	2023
Twenty-Five Twenty-One	2022
Vincenzo	2021
Welcome to Samdal-ri	2023†
When the Weather Is Fine	2020*
Would You Like a Cup of Coffee?	2021
You Are My Spring	2021

Note: The book is based on observing these 88 shows.

*Songs from these shows are included on My Playlist, Appendix 3.

†These shows are discussed in the text, and details are included in Appendix 2.

APPENDIX 2

About the Shows

Business Proposal (사내맞선)

Broadcast: SBS TV, February 28, 2022–April 5, 2022		
Role	**Name**	**Hangul Name**
Writer	Han Seol-hee	한설희 [hansʌɾɯi]
Writer	Hong Bo-hee	홍보희 [hoŋboɯi]
Director	Park Seon-ho	박선호 [paksʌno]
Composer	Park Se-joon	박세준 [paksɛdʑun]

Cast Informtion

Character	**Hangul Name**	**Actor**	**Hangul Name**
Kang Tae-moo	강태무 [kaŋtɛmu]	Ahn Hyo-seop	안효섭 [anjosʌp]
Shin Ha-ri	신하리 [ʃinaɾi]	Kim Se-jeong	김세정 [kimsɛdʑʌŋ]

Captivating the King (세작, 매혹된 자들)

Broadcast: tvN	**January 21 – March 3, 2024**	
Role	**Name**	**Hangul Name**
Writer	Kim Seon-deok	김선덕 [k i m s ʌ n d ʌ k]
Director	Cho Nam-guk	조남국 [tɕ o n a ŋ g u k]
Composer	Park Se-joon	박세준 [p a k s ɛ dʑ u n]

Cast Informtion

Character	**Hangul Name**	**Actor**	**Hangul Name**
Yi In	이인 [i i n]	Jo Jung-suk	조정석 [tɕ o dʑ ʌ ŋ s ʌ k]
Kang Mong-woo	강몽우 [k a ŋ m o ŋ u]	Shin Se-kyung	신세경 [ʃ i n s ɛ g jʌ ŋ]

Crash Landing on You (사랑의 불시착)

Broadcast: SBS TV, February 28, 2022–April 5, 2022		
Role	**Name**	**Hangul Name**
Writer	Park Ji-eun	박지은 [paktʃiɯn]
Director	Lee Jeong-hyo	이정효 [idʑʌŋjo]
Composer	Nam Hye-seung	남혜승 [namjɛsɯŋ]

Cast Information

Character	Hangul Name	Actor	Hangul Name
Ri Jeong-hyeok	리정혁 [lidʑʌŋjʌk]	Hyun Bin	현빈 [hjʌmbin]
Yoon Se-ri	윤세리 [junsɛri]	Son Ye-jin	손예진 [sonjɛdʑin]
Cho Cheol-gang	조철강 [tʃotʃʌlgaŋ]	Oh Man-seok	오만석 [omansʌk]
Master Sergeant Pyo Chi-soo	표치수 [pjotʃisu]	Yang Kyung-won	양경원 [jaŋgjʌŋwʌn]
Sergeant Kim Joo-meok	김주먹 [kimdʑumʌk]	Yoo Su-bin	유수빈 [jaŋgjʌŋwʌn]
Geum Eun-dong	금은동 [kɯmɯndoŋ]	Tang Joon-sang	탕준상 [taŋdʑunsaŋ]
Kim Kwang-beom	김광범 [kiŋgwaŋbʌm]	Lee Shin-young	이신영 [iʃinjʌŋ]
Captain Ri's father/ Ri Chung-ryeol	이충렬 [litʃuŋnjʌl]	Jeon Kuk-hwan	전국환 [tʃʌŋgukhwan]

Dr. Romantic (낭만닥터 김사부)

Broadcast: SBS TV, November 7, 2016–June 17, 2023		
Role	**Name**	**Hangul Name**
Writer	Kang Eun-kyung	강은경 [kaŋɯŋgjʌŋ]
Writer	Lim Hye-min	임혜민 [imjɛmin]
Director	Yoo In-shik	유인식 [juinʃik]
Director	Park Soo-jin	박수진 [paksudʑin]
Director	Lee Gil-bok	이길복 [igilbok]
Director	Kang Bo-sueng	강보승 [kaŋbosɯŋ]
Composer	Jeon Chang-yeop	전창엽 [tɕʌntɕʰaŋjʌp]

Cast Information

Character	Hangul Name	Actor	Hangul Name
Seo Woo-jin	서우진 [sʌudʑin]	Ahn Hyo-seop	안효섭[anjosʌp]
Kim Sabu	김사부 [kimsabu]	Han Suk-kyu	한석규 [hansʌkkju]

Extraordinary Attorney Wu (이상한 변호사 우영우)

Broadcast: ENA, June 29, 2022–August 18, 2022

Role	Name	Hangul Name
Writer	Moon Ji-won	문지원 [mundʑiwʌn]
Director	Yoo In-shik	유인식 [juinʃik]
Composer	Noh Young-shim	노영심 [nojʌŋʃim]

Cast Information

Character	Hangul Name	Actor	Hangul Name
Wu Young-wu	우영우 [ujʌŋu]	Park Eun-bin	박은빈[pagɯmbin]
Lee Jun-ho	이준호 [idʑuno]	Kang Tae-oh	강태오 [kaŋtɛo]

Just Between Lovers (그냥 사랑하는 사이)

Broadcast: JTBC, December 11, 2017–January 18, 2018

Role	Name	Hangul Name
Writer	Yoo Bo-ra	유보라 [jubora]
Director	Kim Jin-won	김진원 [kimdʑinwʌn]
Composer	Nam Hye-seung	남혜승 [namjɛsɯŋ]

Cast Information

Character	Hangul Name	Actor	Hangul Name
Lee Gang-du	이강두 [igaŋdu]	Lee Joon-ho	이준호 [idʑuno]
Ha Mun-su	하문수 [hamunsu]	Won Jin-a	원진아 [wʌndʑina]
Seo Joo-won	서주원 [sʌdʑuwʌn]	Lee Ki-woo	이기우 [igiu]
Jung Yoo-jin	정유진 [tɕʌŋjudʑin]	Kang Han-na	강한나 [kaŋanna]
Sang-man	상만 [saŋman]	Kim Gang-hyun	김강현 [kiŋgaŋjʌn]
Choi Sung-jae	최성재 [tʃwɛsʌŋdʑɛ]	Hong Kyung	홍경 [hoŋgjʌŋ]
Halmoni/Gang-du's grandmother	할머니 [halmʌni]	Na Moon-hee	나문희 [namunɰi]
Ha Mun-su's father/ Ha Dong-chul	하동철 [hadoŋtʃʌl]	Ahn Nae-sang	안내상 [annɛsaŋ]

The King: Eternal Monarch (더 킹: 영원의 군주)

Broadcast: SBS, April 17, 2020–June 12, 2020		
Role	Name	Hangul Name
Writer	Kim Eun-sook	김은숙 [kimɯnsuk]
Director	Baek Sang-hoon	백상훈 [pɛksaŋun]
Director	Yoo Je-won	유제원 [judʑɛwʌn]
Director	Jung Ji-hyun	정지현 [tʃʌŋdʑijʌn]
Composer	Gaemi	개미 [kɛmi]

Cast Information

Character	Hangul Name	Actor	Hangul Name
Lee Gon	이곤 [igon]	Lee Min-ho	이민호 [imino]
Jeong Tae-eul	정태을 [tʃʌŋteɯl]	Kim Go-eun	김고은 [kiŋgoɯn]
Jo-yeong/Jo Eun-sup	조영 [tʃojʌŋ]/조은섭 [tʃoɯnsʌp]	Woo Do-hwan	우도환 [udowan]
Lee Lim	이림 [irim]	Lee Jung-jin	이정진 [idʑʌŋdʑin]
Noh Ok-nam	노옥남 [nooŋnam]	Kim Young-ok	김영옥 [kimjʌŋok]
Kang Sin-jae	강신재 [kaŋʃindʑɛ]	Kim Kyung-nam	김경남 [kiŋgjʌŋnam]
Jeong Tae-eul's father/ Jeong Do-in	정도인 [tʃʌŋdoin]	Jeon Bae-su	전배수 [tʃʌmbɛsu]
Lim Lim's brother/Lee Ho	이호 [io]	Kwon Yool	권율 [kwʌnjul]

The King's Affection (연모)

Broadcast: KBS2, October 11, 2021–December 14, 2021

Role	Name	Hangul Name
Writer	Han Hee-jung	한희정 [hanɰidʑʌŋ]
Director	Song Hyun-wook	송현욱 [soŋjʌnuk]
Director	Lee Hyun-suk	이현숙 [ijʌnsuk]
Composer	Tae-guen	태근 [tɛgɯn]

Cast Information

Character	**Hangul Name**	**Actor Hangul Name**	
Lee Hwi/Dam-i	이휘/담이 [iwi]/[tami]	Park Eun-bin	박은빈 [pagɯmbin]
Jung Ji-un	정지운 [tʃʌŋdʑiun]	Ro Woon	로운 [pagɯmbin]
Prince Lee Hyun	이현 [ijʌn]	Nam Yoon-soo	남윤수 [namjunsu]
Dam-i's grandfather/ Han Ki-jae	한기재 [haŋgidʑɛ]	Yoon Je-moon	윤제문 [jundʑɛmun]
Dam-i's father/King Hyejong	혜종 [hjɛdʑoŋ]	Lee Pil-mo	이필모 [ipilmo]
Dam-i's mother/Bin gung	빈궁 [piŋguŋ]	Han Chae-ah	한채아 [hantʃɛa]
Jung Seok-jo	정석조 [tʃʌŋsʌktʃo]	Bae Soo-bin	배수빈 [pɛsubin]
Court Lady Kim/Kim Sang gung	김상궁 [kimsaŋguŋ]	Baek Hyun-joo	백현주 [pɛkhjʌndʑu]
Eunuch Hong/Hong Naeshi	홍내시 [hoŋnɛʃi]	Ko Kyu-pil	고규필 [kogjupil]
Yoon Hyeong-seol	윤형설 [junjʌŋsʌl]	Kim Jae-chul	김재철 [kimdʑɛtʃʌl]
Shin Young-soo	신영수 [ʃinjʌŋsu]	Park Won-sang	박원상 [pagwʌnsaŋ]

Live Up to Your Name (명불허전)

Broadcast: tvN, August 12, 2017–October 1, 2017

Role	Name	Hangul Name
Writer	Kim Eun-hee	김은희 [kimɯnɰi]
Director	Hong Jong-chan	홍종찬 [hoŋdʑoŋtʃan]
Composer	Various Artists	

Cast Information

Character	Hangul Name	Actor	Hangul Name
Heo Jun	허준 [hʌdʑun]	Eom Hyo-seop	엄효섭 [ʌmjosʌp]
Heo Im	허임 [hʌim]	Kim Nam-gil	김남길[kimnaŋgil]
Choi Yeon-kyung	최연경 [tʃwɛjʌŋgjʌŋ]	Kim Ah-joong	김아중 [kimadʑuŋ]
Dr. Choi Chun-sool	최천술 [tʃwɛtʃʌnsul]	Yoon Joo-sang	유주상 [jundʑusaŋ]
Du-chil	두칠 [tutʃil]	Oh Dae-hwan	오대환 [odɛwan]
Yeon-i	연이 [jʌni]	Shin Rin ah	신린아 [ʃillina]
Dong Mak-gae	동막개 [toŋmakkɛ]	Mun Ka-young	문가영 [muŋgajʌŋ]
Ma Seong-tae	마성태 [masʌŋtɛ]	Kim Myung-gon	김명곤 [kimmjʌŋgon]
The King/King Sunjo	선조 [sʌndʑo]	Jo Seung-yeon	조승연 [tʃosɯŋjʌn]

Misaeng: Incomplete Life (미생 - 아직 살아 있지 못한 자)

Broadcast: tvN, October 17, 2014–December 20, 2014		
Role	Name	Hangul Name
Writer	Jung Yoon-jung	정윤정 [tɕʌŋjundʑʌŋ]
Director	Kim Won-seok	김원석 [kimwʌnsʌk]
Composer	Various Artists	

Cast Information

Character	Hangul Name	Actor	Hangul Name
Jang Geu-rae	장그래 [tɕaŋgɯrɛ]	Im Si-wan	임시완 [imʃiwan]
Park Jong-shik	박종식 [paktɕoŋʃik]	Kim Hee-won	김희원 [kimɰiwʌn]

Mr. Queen (철인왕후)

Broadcast: tvN, December 12, 2020–February 14, 2021		
Role	Name	Hangul Name
Writer	Park Gye-ok	박계옥 [pakkjɛok]
Writer	Choi Ah-il	최아일 [tɕʰwɛail]
Director	Yoon Sung-sik	윤성식 [junsʌŋʃik]
Composer	Various Artists	

Cast Information

Character	Hangul Name	Actor	Hangul Name
Jang Bong-hwan	장봉환 [tɕaŋboŋwan]	Choi Jin-hyuk	최진혁 [tɕʰwɛdʑinjʌk]
Kim So-yong	김소용 [kimsojoŋ]	Shin Hye-sun	신혜선 [ʃinjɛsʌn]

Navillera (나빌레라)

Broadcast: tvN, March 22, 2021–April 27, 2021		
Role	Name	Hangul Name
Writer	Lee Seun-mi	이은미 [iɯmmi]
Director	Han Dong-hwa	한동화 [handoŋwa]
Composer	Various Artists	

Cast Information

Character	Hangul Name	Actor	Hangul Name
Shim Deok-chul	심덕철 [ʃimdʌktʃʌl]	Park In-hwan	박인환 [paginwan]
Lee Chae-rok	이채록 [itʃɛrok]	Song Kang	송강 [soŋgaŋ]

Once Upon a Small Town (어쩌다 전원일기)

Broadcast: Kakao TV, September 5, 2022–September 28, 2022		
Role	Name	Hangul Name
Writer	Baek Eun-kyeong	백은경 [pɛgɯngjʌŋ]
Director	Kwon Seok-jang	권석장 [kwʌnsʌktɕaŋ]
Composer	Moon Seong-nam	문석남 [munsʌŋnam]

Cast Information

Character	Hangul Name	Actor	Hangul Name
Han Ji-yool	한지율 [handʑijul]	Choo Young-woo	추영우 [tʃujʌŋu]
Ahn Ja-young	안자영 [andʑaŋjʌŋ]	Park Soo-young	박수영 [paksujʌŋ]
Lee Sang-hyeon	이상현 [isaŋjʌn]	Baek Sung-chul	백성철[pɛksʌŋtɕʰʌl]

Prison Playbook (슬기로운 감빵생활)

Broadcast: tvN, November 22, 2017–January 18, 2018

Role	Name	Hangul Name
Writer	Jung Bo-hoon	정보훈 [tɕʌŋboun]
Writer	Lee Woo-jung	이우정 [iudʑʌŋ]
Director	Shin Won-ho	신원호 [ʃinwʌno]
Composer	Old Standards	

Cast Information

Character	Hangul Name	Actor	Hangul Name
Kim Je-hyeok	김제혁 [kimdʑɛjʌk]	Park Hae-soo	박해수 [pakɛsu]
Kim Ji-ho	김지호 [kimdio]	Krystal Jung	정수정 [tɕʌŋsudʑʌŋ]
Lee Joon-ho	이준호 [idʑuno]	Jung Kyoung-ho	정경호 [tʃʌŋgjʌŋo]
Lee Joon-dol	이준돌 [idʑundol]	Kim Kyung-nam	김형남 [kimjʌŋnam]
Jean Valjean	장발장 [tɕaŋbaldʑaŋ]	Kang Seung-yoon	강승윤 [kaŋsɯŋjun]
Kim Min-cheol	김민철 [kimmintʃʌl]	Choi Moo-sung	최무성 [tʃwɛmusʌŋ]
Errand Boy/Soji	소지 [sodʑi]	Kim Han-jong	김한종 [kimandʑoŋ]
Jailbird/Kim Young-chul	김영철 [kimjʌŋtʃʌl]	Kim Sung-cheol	김성철 [kimsʌŋtʃʌl]
Professor Myung	명교수 [mjʌŋgjosu]	Jung Jae-sung	정재성 [tʃʌŋdʑɛsʌŋ]
Gangster/Gal Dae-bong	갈대봉 [kaldɛboŋ]	Lee Ho-cheol	이호철 [iotʃʌl]
Crony, Dong-ho	동호 [toŋo]	Ahn Chang-hwan	안창환 [antʃaŋwan]

Romance Is a Bonus Book (로맨스는 별책부록)

Broadcast: tvN, January 26, 2019–March 17, 2019

Role	Name	Hangul Name
Writer	Jung Hyun-jung	정현정 [tʃʌŋjʌndʑʌŋ]
Director	Lee Jung-hyo	이정효 [idʑʌŋjo]
Composer	Nam Hye-seung	남혜승 [namjɛsɯŋ]
Composer	Jeon Jong-hyuk	전종혁 [tʃʌndʑoŋjʌk]
Composer	Park Sang-hye	박상혜 [paksaŋjɛ]
Composer	Go Eun-jong	고은종 [koɯndʑoŋ]

Cast Information

Character	Hangul Name	Actor	Hangul Name
Kang Dan-i	강단이 [kaŋdani]	Lee Na-young	이나영 [inajʌŋ]
Cha Eun-ho	차은호 [tʃaɯno]	Lee Jong-suk	이종석 [idʑoŋsʌk]
Director Go Yu-seon	고유선 감독 [kojusʌŋgamdok]	Kim Yu-mi	김유미 [kimjumi]
Song Hae-rin	송해린 [soŋɛrin]	Jung Eugen	정유진 [tʃʌŋjudʑin]
President Kim Jae-min	김재민 사장 [kimdʑɛminsadʑaŋ]	Kim Tae-woo	김태우 [kimtɛu]

Welcome to Samdal-ri (웰컴투 삼달리)

Broadcast: JTBC, December 2, 2023–January 21, 2024

Role	Name	Hangul Name
Writer	Kwon Hye-joo	권혜주 [kwinjɛdʑu]
Director	Cha Young-hoon	차영훈 [tʃajʌŋun]
Composer	Various Artists	

Cast Information

Character	Hangul Name	Actor	Hangul Name
Cho Sam-dal	조삼달 [tʃosamdal]	Shin Hye-sun	신혜선 [ʃinjɛsʌn]
Cho Yong-pil	조용필 [tʃojoŋpil]	Ji Chang-wook	지창욱 [tʃitʃaŋuk]

Note: I worked closely with Stefan Gehrman and Professor Kyla Park, my Korean teacher, to make this table. Stefan made the original table, collecting basic information from Wikipedia about each of the shows. I turned to Professor Park to sort out the English spelling of Korean names. For example, 우 might be written "Oo" or "Wu." She proposed that we show each name using the International Phonetic Alphabet. This could save English speakers from some important mispronunciations. For example, I thought "Hyun Bin" would be pronounced "High-un Bin." I learned that "Hyun" is one syllable, not two, and had to practice the quiet sound of the opening "h." It was the same for "Heo Im": I thought it was "Hay-o Im," but "Heo" is also one syllable. "Eo" is not pronounced "e-o," in two syllables, but as one sound, which is close to "gnaw." Food for thought!

Sources:
Wikipedia, Business Proposal; NamuWikiWiki, 사내 맞선(드라마)
Wikipedia, Captivating the King; NamuWiki, 세작, 매혹된 자들
Wikipedia, Crash Landing on You; NamuWikiWiki, 사랑의 불시착

Wikipedia, Dr. Romantic; NamuWiki, 낭만닥터 김사부
Wikipedia, Extraordinary Attorney Wu; NamuWiki, 이상한 변호사 우영우
Wikipedia, Just between Lovers; NamuWiki, 그냥 사랑하는 사이
Wikipedia, The King: Eternal Monarch; NamuWiki, 더 킹: 영원의 군주
Wikipedia, The King's Affection; NamuWiki, 연모
Wikipedia, Live Up to Your Name; NamuWiki, 명불허전(드라마)
Wikipedia, Misaeng; NamuWiki, 미생(드라마)
Wikipedia, Mr. Queen; Namuwiki, 철인왕후(드라마)
Wikipedia, Navilera; NamuWiki, 나빌레라(드라마)
Wikipedia, Once Upon a Small Town; NamuWiki, 어쩌다 전원일기
Wikipedia, Prison Playbook; NamuWiki, 슬기로운 감빵생활
Wikipedia, Romance Is a Bonus Book; NamuWiki, 로맨스는 별책부록
Wikipedia, Welcome to Sandal-ri; NamuWiki, 웰컴투 삼달리

APPENDIX 3

My Original Soundtrack Playlist

Table A.3 My Playlist

Show	Song	Artist(s)	Writer(s)
The Bride of Habaek	Glass Bridge	Savina & Drones	Nam Hye-seung, MIYO, Jello Ann
The Bride of Habaek	Reminds Me Of	Junggigo	Nam Hye-seung, Park Jin-ho
The Bride of Habaek	The Reason Why	Yang Da-il	Nam Hye-seung, Park Jin-ho, Glody, Poly
Chocolate	You & I	Ha Ji-won & Yoon Kye-sang	Jung Ye-kyung, ID:Earth
Cinderella and the Four Knights	My Romeo	Jessi	Kim Yu-kyung, Oh Joon-sung
Cinderella and the Four Knights	Stars Fall on You	Dickpunks	Kim Yu-kyung, Oh Joon-sung
Crash Landing on You	Flower	Yoon Mi-rae	Nam Hye-seung, Park Jin-ho, Surf Green
Crash Landing on You	Here I Am Again	Yerin Baek	Nam Hye-seung, Surf Green
Crash Landing on You	Let Us Go	Crush	Dong Woo-seok, Yoo Jung-hyun, Jayins
Crash Landing on You	The Hill of Yearning	April 2nd	Nam Hye-seung, Kim Kyung-hee
Crash Landing on You	When That Day Comes	Instrumental	Nam Hye-seung, Park Sang-hee
Goblin: The Lonely and Great God	Beautiful	Crush	Lee Seung-ju, Hwang Chan-hee, Jihoon
Hometown Cha-Cha-Cha	Wish	Choi Yu-ree	Choi Yu-ree

Show	Song	Artist(s)	Writer(s)
Hospital Playlist 1	In Front of City Hall at the Subway Station	Kwak Jin-eon	Kim Chang-gi
Hospital Playlist 1	Lonely Night	Kwon Jin-ah	Kim Tae-won
Hospital Playlist 1	Me to You, You to Me	Mido and Falasol	Song Bong-joo
Hospital Playlist 2	In Front of the Post Office in Autumn	Kim Dae-myeung	Kim Hyun-sung
Hospital Playlist 2	Superstar	Mido and Falasol	Lee Han-chul
Just Between Lovers	Aurora	Savina & Drones (with Kim Kyung-hee)	Nam Hye-seung, Kim Kyung-hee, Jello Ann, Park Sang-hee
Just Between Lovers	Just Because	Ra.D	Nam Hye-seung, Park Jin-ho
Just Between Lovers	Just Between Lovers Title	Elaine	Nam Hye-seung, Park Sang-hee, Jello Ann
Just between Lovers	True Love	Lee Jun-ho	Nam Hye-seung, Park Jin-ho
The King: Eternal Monarch	Gravity	Kim Jong Wan	Ra.L, Naomi, Gaemi
The King: Eternal Monarch	I Fall in Love	Ha Sung-woon	Noheul, Gaemi, KRAZY PARK
The King: Eternal Monarch	Maze	Yongzoo	Ogya, Charles, Gaemi
The King: Eternal Monarch	Orbit	Hwasa	Park Woo-sang, Sora
The King's Affection	If I	Baek Z Young	VIP
King the Land	Eyes, Nose, Lips	Taeyang	Teddy Park, Taeyang
Misaeng	Fly	Yi Sung Yol	Park A-sel
Mr. Queen	Bong Hwan A	Norazo	Jong Young-soo, Cheon Woo-kyung, Kang Seung-ho, Choi Soo-hyuk
My Liberation Notes	Be My Birthday	Ha Hyun-sang	Naiv, 9duck
My Liberation Notes	My Liberation Notes	Choe Jeong-in	Choe Jeong-in

Show	Song	Artist(s)	Writer(s)
One Spring Night	Is It You	Rachael Yamagata	Rachael Yamagata, Lee Nam-yeon, Kevin Salem
One Spring Night	No Direction	Rachael Yamagata	Lee Nam-yeon, Kevin Salem, Rachael Yamagata
One Spring Night	Spring Rain	Oscar Dunbar	Lee Nam-yeon, Kevin Salem, Rachael Yamagata
Our Blues	For Love	10CM	Jihoon, Lee Seung-ju, Choi In-hwan
Our Blues	Happy Song	MeloMance	Jihoon, Lee Seung-ju, Choi In-hwan
Our Blues	Once Again	Winter & Ningning	Viktoria Hansen, Kirat Singh, Mich Hansen, Jacob Uchorczak, Jihoon
Our Blues	Only You	Choi Seong-geun & Kim Ji-soo	Choi Seong-geun, Kim Ji-soo
Our Blues	With You	Jimin & Ha Sung-woon	Jihoon, Rocoberry
Prison Playbook	Bravo, My Life!	SSaW	Kim Jong-jin
Prison Playbook	Goodbye Now	015B	Jung Seok-won
Prison Playbook	Unfortunate Guy	Kim Kwang-seok	Kim Eui-chul
Prison Playbook	Snail	Panic	Lee Juck
Romance Is a Bonus Book	All I Do	Roy Kim	Kim Sang-woo, Nam Hye-seung, Park Jin-ho
Romance Is a Bonus Book	Happy End	SAya & Kim Ki-won	Nam Hye-seung, Surf Green
Rookie Historian: Gu Rae Hyung	My Dream	Yoon Mi-rae	Lee Na-young, Kanasus Brew, Naeun
Touch Your Heart	What If Love	Wendy	Baek Chan, DJ Kayvon
When the Weather Is Fine	Doors of Time	Jung Yup	Banana, March, Clef Crew, Park Jang-hyun
When the Weather Is Fine	Like a Winter's Dream	Kwak Jin-eon	Jeong Joong-han
When the Weather Is Fine	Moody Night	Jeon Sang-keun	KZ, Who's H, Jung Soo-min, Clef Crew, Banana, March, Yoo Sang-gyun
You Are My Spring	Dear My Spring	Onew	Lee Mina, Yoon Young-jun
You Are My Spring	Still Wonder	Ha Hyun-sang	Naiv, 9duck

Sources: Apple Music, cross-checked with the Google AI search engine and www.melon.com.

Notes

Acknowledgments

1. Korean names typically have three syllables, with the family name first, followed by the two-syllable first name. In representing these names in English, people make choices about the romanization of the Hangul and the order of the family and first names. I tried to present names as people stated, so the order of names and the spelling vary according to the person's preferences. I suggest, for ease of reading this book, that one use the set of names as the name and put aside issues of first and last.

Introduction

1. Fullilove, "Orange Park."
2. Thompson, "National Negro Labor Council."
3. Thompson and Thompson, *Homeboy Came to Orange.*
4. Fullilove, *Root Shock.*
5. Wikipedia, "Heo Im." And maybe *the* greatest! The "who's the greatest" conversation is vivid in sports. In 2025, a group of statisticians announced a method to account for history and find who was the "greatest" in baseball. It turned out to be Barry Bonds, not Babe Ruth. Nazaryan, "Bonds."
6. Fullilove, *Root Shock*, p. 10.
7. Ling, The Dao of World Politics, p. 49.
8. Wikipedia, "Mr. Queen."
9. Shankman, "Cumberland Divided."

Chapter 1

1. Alexander et al., *A Pattern Language.*
2. My exposition of the stories will be indented for clarity.
3. Brittanica, "Go Game."
4. Lucas, "Date of the Exodus."
5. Bishop, "Street by Street."
6. Jenkins, Bedrock.

Chapter 2

1. Sullivan, "Town Shrink."
2. Puett and Gross-Loh, *The Path.*
3. Puett and Gross-Loh, *The Path*, p. 60.
4. Ames and Hall, *Dao De Jing*, p. 39.
5. Puett and Gross-Loh, *The Path*, p. 69.
6. Puett and Gross-Loh, *The Path*, p. 72.
7. Puett and Gross-Loh, *The Path*, p. 166.
8. Puett and Gross-Loh, *The Path*, p. 166.
9. Mao, *On Contradiction.*
10. Johnson, personal communication.
11. Wells, "Microaggressions."

12. Laughter, "Toward a Theory of Micro-kindness."
13. Rohr, "Possessed by the Wrong Perspective."
14. A colleague pointed out that in 1944, high school students in East Orange, New Jersey, started the "candy stripers" by sewing bright uniforms and volunteering at East Orange General Hospital. Wikipedia, "Hospital Volunteers." A photo of me at that demonstration was in *The New York Times.*
15. Kleinman has written numerous books on this topic, but two of great importance for this book are *What Really Matters* and *The Soul of Care.*
16. Kleinman, *What Really Matters*, p. 208 (emphasis added).
17. Barker, *Regeneration*; MacKinnon, *Regeneration.*
18. Owen, *Dulce et Decorum Est.* This quotation is from the Roman poet Horace and is translated as: Sweet and fitting it is to die for one's country.
19. Wilson, "Dr W. H. R. Rivers."
20. Here's a thought experiment: imagine a blast explodes in the middle of the web of relationships. What are the bridges—in Dr. Paul Browde's sense—that will need to be rebuilt?
21. Wikipedia, "Poong."
22. Wikipedia, "My Liberation Notes."
23. Ginger and Christiano, *Cold War Against Labor*, see especially pp. 346–373; Thompson, *The National Negro Labor Council.*

Chapter 3

1. Wikipedia, "Heo Im."
2. *Alcoholics Anonymous.*
3. Wikipedia, "Heo Jun."
4. Wikipedia, "Navillera."

Chapter 4

1. Hughes, "Theme for English."
2. Spotify, "Powerdance." In Appendix 3, you will find my playlist of favorite songs from K-dramas.
3. If you missed this Oscar-winning film, it is a complex story of three families, one rich, two poor. It is worth your time! The Korean's insights are useful. The Korean, "The Forgotten Neoliberal Man."
4. Erickson and Vosburg, *Betrayed by Work.*
5. Fullilove et al, "Task-Oriented Group."
6. Nelson, "Steel Drivin' Man."
7. Hong, "South Korean TV."
8. Lyrics Translate, "Happy End (English Ver.) Lyrics."
9. Lyrics Translate, "Happy End Lyrics" (Korean version).
10. Simmons, personal communication.
11. Kimchi Mamas, "Oori" (emphasis added).
12. Garrison, "Just know."

Chapter 5

1. Grumet, Anthony F. C. Wallace, p. 178.
2. Grumet, *Anthony F. C. Wallace*, p. 182.
3. Grumet, *Anthony F. C. Wallace*, p. 182.
4. Grumet, *Anthony F. C. Wallace*, p. 185.
5. Kwon, "Author R.O. Kwon's Guide to Seoul."
6. Visit Korea, "Seodaemun Prison."
7. War and Women's Human Rights Museum, "About Us."

8. Korea Clickers, "Jangheung Prison."
9. Wallace and Fullilove, *Collective Consciousness*.
10. I've observed and written about the delays in response to several epidemics, including the AIDS epidemic: Morales and Fullilove, "'Many Are Called . . .'"; the crack epidemic: Watkins, Fullilove, and Fullilove, "Arms Against Illness"; and the COVID pandemic: Jirmanus et al., "Too Many Deaths."
11. Rosman, "He Was One of the Central Park Five."
12. Prevost, "Sylvia Ryerson's Calls."
13. Prinz, "Speech."

Chapter 6

1. On Netflix, this show is called *Rain or Shine*. I find *Just Between Lovers* both more informative and closer to the title in Korean. *Rain or Shine* is taken from the name of the ice cream shop where the protagonists are standing at the time of the collapse. We see the name on a fragment of the shop window in the rubble where the youths are trapped.
2. VarietyRecaps, "Just Between Lovers Recaps, Episodes 1–16," Episode 2.
3. VarietyRecaps, "Just Between Lovers Recaps, Episodes 1–16," Episode 6.
4. VarietyRecaps, "Just Between Lovers Recaps, Episodes 1–16," Episode 6 (emphasis in original).
5. Paul Browde, personal communication.
6. VarietyRecaps, "Just Between Lovers Recaps, Episodes 1–16," Episode 6.
7. Drew Jackson, "Morning Sit Manuscript," May 20, 2025, personal communication.
8. Cumings, *Korea's Place in the Sun*, p. 301.
9. Wallace et al., "Deindustrialization."
10. Cumings, *Korea's Place in the Sun*, p. 341.
11. Ringen et al., *Korean State*.
12. Wikipedia, "Aging of South Korea."
13. Chao and Gooch, "The Country with the World's Worst Drink Problem."
14. Yoon, "Suicide."
15. Jung, "Sampoong."
16. Korea Herald, "2014 Ferry Disaster."
17. Lee, "Itaewon Tragedy."
18. Kim, *Homebrewed Christianity Guide*, p. 166; Ko, "Broken Heart," 2017. Her case study of a woman with *han* underscores both the complexity of what is meant by *han* and the need for movement of Spirit to get out of that state.
19. Kim, *Homebrewed Christianity Guide*, p. 172.
20. Maryland Lynching Memorial, "Bryan Stevenson Quote."

Chapter 7

1. Wikipedia, "The King's Affection."
2. Ames and Hall, *Dao De Jing*, p. 160. The authors note that use of *dao* in two senses is a pun, in which the first means "robbers" and the second means "righteous."
3. In South Korea, teachers and others can give someone a second or third name as a mark of admiration.
4. Ellis, "The Arc of the Moral Universe."
5. Ellis, "The Arc of the Moral Universe."
6. Buehrens, Transcendentalists.
7. Manker-Seale, "Moral Arc."
8. Manker-Seale, "Moral Arc."
9. Manker-Seale, "Moral Arc."
10. Yasir, "Where 'No One Wanted Girls.'"

11. BlackPast, "(1955) Martin Luther King Jr."
12. The king in *Captivating the King* is able to do this, confounding his enemies over and over. He plays Go.
13. Baker, "From Scorn to Respect."
14. Wallace, Carl von Clausewitz.
15. SailorJumun, "The King's Affection."
16. Hong, *Birth of the Korean Cool*, p. 70.
17. Erikson, *Everything in Its Path*, pp. 187–188.
18. Kutcher, "The Fifth Relationship."
19. Vadukul, "The Unlikely Friendship."

Chapter 8

1. Bullen, "Are There 3, 5, 7, 9 or 36 Different Plot Types?"
2. Quote Investigator, "There Are Only Two Plots."
3. I was startled to read in the Dramabeans recap that she says this in English, which I had never noticed.
4. Rennis, "We Have a Situation Here!"; Ballestero, "We Have a Situation Here!"
5. Polti, *The Thirty-Six Dramatic Situations.*
6. Merriam-Webster, "Athleisure Wear." This is defined as "casual clothing designed to be worn both for exercising and for general use." They offer an example: "'Of course, *athleisure* has lately become a fashion buzzword, a term intended to embrace the kind of clothing that a woman might be able to wear at work, to the gym, and then to dinner.'—Rob Haskell." We could add that she could wear it to North Korea!
7. Cho et al., *Integrated Korean*, p. 43.
8. LollyPip, "Crash Landing on You: Episode 1."
9. Cumings, *Korea's Place in the Sun*, pp. 186–187.
10. Stack, "Korean War."
11. Kuzmarov, "Korean War."
12. Cachero, "Korean Orphans."
13. Matray, "Korean War 101."
14. Situation Analysis Class, *One Step Can't Hurt.*
15. I feel the same way and do the same things. It is hard to express the delight I felt when I got to Korea and was able to see in real life what I'd gotten to know via television.
16. Schmitt and Klein, "Fighting in the Fog."
17. It was a great moment in my study of the Korean language when I realized this!
18. Yoon Se-ri also builds a posse with the women of the village, a process my colleagues and I addressed in a separate paper. Maruyama, "The Laundry and the DMZ."
19. Zuckerman, "Are We in a New Golden Age for the Movie Soundtrack?"
20. Wikipedia, "Crash Landing on You."
21. Lyrics Translate, "Hill of Yearning."
22. Jenkins, "Bedrock," p. 27.
23. Bunche, "Some Reflections on Peace in Our Time."
24. Heon-Klin, "The Influence of Geopolitical Change on the Well-Being of a Population."

Chapter 9

1. Ó Tuama, *50 Poems*, p. 66.
2. Carroll, *Alice's Adventures in Wonderland*, pp. 2–3.
3. Brunette, "'The King, the Eternal Monarch' Time Stop."
4. MacGyver, Pilot. It turns out oral surgeons do magic with paperclips as well. Merriam-Webster, "MacGyver."

5. Hong, *The Power of Nunchi.*
6. Fullilove, "Psychiatric Implications of Displacement," p. 1522.
7. Coles, *Children of Crisis*, p. 365.

Chapter 10

3. Wikipedia, "Because This Is My First Life."
4. Porter, *Pollyanna. Alcoholics Anonymous*: Although the so-called Big Book of Alcoholics Anonymous has no "author," it was largely written by Bill Wilson. Beck, "Cognitive Therapy."
5. Havel, "Disturbing the Peace," pp. 181–182.
6. Havel, "Disturbing the Peace," pp. 181–182.
7. Bourgeault, *Mystical Hope.*
8. Kim, The Homebrewed Christianity Guide.
9. Fullilove, *Root Shock*, p. 101.
10. K-drama takes a different perspective from that of Yoda, who famously instructed, "There is no try, do or don't do."
11. Shakespeare, "The Complete works of William Shakespeare."
12. Hong, *The Power of Nunchi*, p. 17. The number of invasions may be lower or higher than this number without changing the implication that Koreans had to learn how to survive and rebuild, and it is this knowledge that they are sharing with us.
13. Bell, "Cultivating Resiliency in Youth." Psychiatrist Carl Bell, who was a martial artist working in inner-city Chicago, proposed the term "heart" to mean "indomitable fighting spirit" and saw the development of "heart" as a key to resiliency in youth.

Bibliography

Alcoholics Anonymous: The Story of How Many Thousands of Men and Women Have Recovered from Alcoholism. New York: Alcoholics Anonymous World Services, 2002.

Alexander, Christopher, Sara Ishikawa, and Murray Silverstein. *A Pattern Language: Towns, Buildings, Construction*. New York: Oxford University Press, 1977.

Ames, Roger T., and David L. Hall, trans. *Dao De Jing "Making This Life Significant": A Philosophical Translation*. New York: Ballantine Books, 2003.

Anisa, Hellcat, Sunny, and LollyPip. "Live Up to Your Name." Dramabeans recaps, accessed June 20, 2025, https://dramabeans.com/shows/live-up-to-your-name/.

"Athleisure Wear." *Merriam-Webster Dictionary*, last modified June 17, 2025, https://www.merriam-webster.com/dictionary/athleisure#:~:text=%3A%20casual%20clothing%20designed%20to%20be,exercising%20and%20for%20general%20use.

Ballestero, Martyn. "We Have a Situation Here!" *The Ballestero Blog*, February 18, 2013, http://martynballestero.com/2013/02/18/we-have-a-situation-here/.

Baker, Peter. "From Scorn to Respect, Carter's Legacy Evolved After His Presidency." *The New York Times*, December 29, 2024, https://www.nytimes.com/2024/12/29/us/politics/jimmy-carter-legacy-presidency.html.

Barker, Pat. *Regeneration*. New York: Viking Press, 1991.

Beck, Aaron T. "Cognitive Therapy: Past, Present, and Future." *Journal of Consulting and Clinical Psychology* 61, no. 2 (1993): 194–198.

Bell, Carl C. "Cultivating Resiliency in Youth." *Journal of Adolescent Health* 29, no. 5 (2001): 375–381.

Bishop, Mary. "Street by Street Block by Block: How Urban Renewal Uprooted Black Roanoke." *Roanoke Times and World News Special Section*, January 29, 1995.

BlackPast. "(1955) Martin Luther King Jr., 'The Montgomery Bus Boycott,'" January 17, 2012, https://www.blackpast.org/african-american-history/1955-martin-luther-king-jr-montgomery-bus-boycott/.

Booker, Christopher. *The Seven Basic Plots: Why We Tell Stories*. London: Bloomsbury Academic, 2006.

Bosman, Fred, Henk Bakker, and Mindy Thompson Fullilove. "Mental Health Center in Post-Disaster Recovery: Ten-Year Retrospective of Mediant's Work in Enschede, Netherlands." *International Journal of Mental Health* 42, no. 2–3 (2013): 130–148.

Bourgeault, Cynthia. *Mystical Hope: Trusting in the Mercy of God*. Boston: Cowley Publications, 2001.

Braceland, Lawrence C., and Marsha L. Dutton. *Spiritual Friendship*. Trappist, KY: Cistercian Publications, 2010.

Britannica. "Go Board Game," last updated April 14, 2025, https://www.britannica.com/topic/go-game.

Brunette. "'The King: Eternal Monarch' Time Stop: How Does Lee Gon Measure the Duration of a Time Stop?" *ThreadReader*, May 24, 2020, https://threadreaderapp.com/thread/1264739646249951233.html#:~:text=Equivalently%2C%20the%20duration%20of%20a,square%20of%20a%20prime%20number.&text=Here%20is%20a%20list%20of,mentioned%20about%20in%20episode%2011.

Bullen, Emma. "Are There 3, 5, 7, 9 or 36 Different Plot Types? [The Definitive Answer]." *Medium*, accessed June 20, 2025, https://medium.com/nicely-said/are-there-3-5-7-9-or-36-different-plot-types-the-definitive-answer-nicely-said-90db2a60d4df#:~:text=If%20you%20have%20a%20quick,Georges%20Polti's%2036%20Dramatic%20Situations.

Bunche, Ralph. "Some Reflections on Peace in Our Time." Nobel Prize Lecture, December 11, 1950, accessed December 9, 2025, https://www.nobelprize.org/prizes/peace/1950/bunche/lecture/.

Cachero, Paulina. "Korean Orphans Languish in System as Tradition, New Laws Make Adoption Difficult." *The Groundtruth Project*, July 20, 2019, https://thegroundtruthproject.org/korean-orphans-languish-system-tradition-new-laws-make-adoption-difficult/.

Carroll, Lewis. *Alice's Adventures in Wonderland*. Boston: Lee and Shepard, 1869.

Chang, Jeanie Y. *How K-Dramas Can Transform Your Life: Powerful Lessons on Belongingness, Healing and Mental Health*. Hoboken, NJ: Wiley, 2024.

Chao, Steve, and Liz Gooch. "The Country with the World's Worst Drink Problem." *Al Jazeera*, February 7, 2016, https://www.aljazeera.com/features/2016/2/7/the-country-with-the-worlds-worst-drink-problem.

Charon, Rita, Sayantani Das Gupta, Nellie Hermann, Craig Irvine, Eric R. Marcus, Edgar Rivera Colon, Danielle Spencer, and Maura Spiegel. *The Principles and Practice of Narrative Medicine*. New York: Oxford University Press, 2017.

Cho, Young-mee, Hyo Sang Lee, Carol Schulz, Ho-Min Sohn, and Sung-Ock Sohn. *Integrated Korean: Beginning 2*. Honolulu: University of Hawaii Press, 2010.

Christie, Agatha. *A Murder Is Announced*. New York: Black Dog & Leventhal Publishers, 2006.

Chung, Chai-sik. *Korean Tradition of Religion, Society, and Ethics: A Comparative and Historical Self-Understanding and Looking Beyond*. New York: Routledge, 2017.

Coles, Robert. *Children of Crisis, Volume 1*. Boston: Little Brown & Co., 1967.

Collectsfallenstars. "Gravity: A Summary of the Development of Jeong TaeEul's Feelings for Lee Gon in 'The King: Eternal Monarch.' Analysis in 3 Parts," accessed July 2, 2024, https://collectsfallenstars.tumblr.com/archive.

Collectsfallenstars. "In Defense of Kim Eun Sook's 'The King: Eternal Monarch,'" accessed July 2, 2024, https://www.tumblr.com/collectsfallenstars/618670458117701632/warning-absolutely-long-post-in-defense-of-kim?source=share.

Collectsfallenstars. "Lee Gon's 3 Rules and How and When He Fell in Love with Jeong TaeEul: An Analysis in 2 Parts," accessed July 2, 2024, https://collectsfallenstars.tumblr.com/archive.
Cumings, Bruce. *The Korean War: A History.* New York: Modern Library, 2011.
Cumings, Bruce. *Korea's Place in the Sun: A Modern History.* New York: W. W. Norton, 1997.
Cumings, Bruce. *North Korea: Another Country.* New York: The New Press, 2011.
Downs, Jim. *Maladies of Empire.* Boston: Harvard University Press, 2023.
Dramallama, Drama Geek, KdramaJen, Kmuse, and Karie the Maknae. "Prison Playbook." Dramabeans recaps, accessed June 15, 2025, https://dramabeans.com/2017/11/smart-prison-living-episode-1/.
Elflein, John. "Percentage of U.S. Cigarette Smokers 1965–2019." *Statista,* September 18, 2024, https://www.statista.com/statistics/184418/percentage-of-cigarette-smoking-in-the-us/.
Ellis, Deborah. "The Arc of the Moral Universe Is Long, but It Bends Toward Justice." *The White House: President Barack Obama Blog,* October 21, 2011, https://obamawhitehouse.archives.gov/blog/2011/10/21/arc-moral-universe-long-it-bends-toward-justice#:~:text=Martin%20Luther%20King%2C%20Jr.%2C,time%2C%20but%20it%20does%20happen.
Erickson, Julia, and Suzanne Vosburg. *Betrayed by Work: Women's Stories of Trauma, Healing and Hope After Being Fired.* Coral Gables: Mango Publishing Group, 2021.
Erikson, Kai T. *Everything in Its Path: Destruction of Community in the Buffalo Creek Flood.* New York: Simon and Schuster, 1976.
Feng, Gia-fu, and Jane English, trans. *Tao Te Ching.* New York: Vintage Books, 1989.
Ferdman, Roberto A. "South Koreans Drink Twice as Much Liquor as Russians and More Than Four Times as Much as Americans." *Quartz,* last updated July 21, 2022, https://qz.com/171191/south-koreans-drink-twice-as-much-liquor-as-russians-and-more-than-four-times-as-much-as-americans.
French, David. "'The Bear' and the Need for a Place to Belong." *The New York Times,* July 16, 2023, https://www.nytimes.com/2023/07/16/opinion/the-bear-fx.html.
Fullilove, Mindy Thompson. "The Ecology of Inequality," filmed October 27, 2017, at TEDxMidAtlantic, Washington, DC, video, 12:19, https://www.ted.com/talks/mindy_fullilove_the_ecology_of_inequality.
Fullilove, Mindy Thompson. *Main Street: How a City's Heart Connects Us All.* New York: New Village Press, 2020.
Fullilove, Mindy Thompson. "Orange Park and the Making of Attachment," in *Olmsted Trees* by Stanley Greenberg, Munich: Hirmer Publishers, 2022, pp. 81–87.
Fullilove, Mindy Thompson. "Psychiatric Implications of Displacement: Contributions from the Psychology of Place." *American Journal of Psychiatry* 153 (1996): 1516–1523.
Fullilove, Mindy Thompson. *Root Shock: How Tearing Up City Neighborhoods Hurts America, and What We Can Do About It.* New York: New Village Press, 2016.
Fullilove, Mindy Thompson. *Urban Alchemy: Restoring Joy in America's Sorted-Out Cities.* New York: New Village Press, 2013.

Fullilove, Mindy Thompson, Lourdes Hernandez-Cordero, Jennifer Stevens Madoff, and Robert E. Fullilove III. "Promoting Collective Recovery Through Organizational Mobilization: The Post-9/11 Disaster Relief Work of NYC RECOVERS." *Journal of Biosocial Science* 36, no. 4 (2004): 479–489.

Fullilove, Mindy Thompson, Olga Pacheco, and Chrystal Fourchard. "Task-Oriented Group in a Day Hospital." *Journal of the National Medical Association* 77, no. 12 (1985): 995–998.

Garrison, Drew. "Just know." *Twitter*, June 19, 2024, https://x.com/DrewGarrison/status/1803561281460297888.

Ginger, Ann Fagan, and David Christiano, eds. *The Cold War Against Labor.* Berkeley, CA: Meiklejohn Civil Liberties Institute, 1987.

Glanz, James, and Campbell Robertson. "Lockdown Delays Cost at Least 36,000 Lives, Data Show." *The New York Times*, May 22, 2020, https://www.nytimes.com/2020/05/20/us/coronavirus-distancing-deaths.html.

"Go Game." *Britannica*, accessed March 10, 2024, https://www.britannica.com/topic/go-game.

Grumet, Robert S, ed. *Anthony F. C. Wallace: Revitalizations and Mazeways, Essays on Culture Change, Volume 1.* Lincoln: University of Nebraska Press, 2003.

Han, Kang. *Human Acts*, translated by Deborah Smith. London: Granta Books, 2020.

Havel, Vaclav. "Disturbing the Peace." Vaclav Havel Center, accessed April 7, 2026, https://havelcenter.org/2015/05/04/disturbing-the-peace/?utm_source=substack&utm_medium=email.

Héon-Klin, Véronique, Erika Sieber, Julia Huebner, and Mindy Thompson Fullilove. "The Influence of Geopolitical Change on the Well-Being of a Population: The Berlin Wall." *American Journal of Public Health* 91, no. 3 (2001): 369–374.

Herman, Judith. *Truth and Repair: How Trauma Survivors Envision Justice.* New York: Basic Books, 2024.

Hoff, Benjamin. *The Tao of Pooh.* London: Farshore, 2022.

Hong, Euny. *The Birth of the Korean Cool: How One Nation Is Conquering the World Through Pop Culture.* New York: Picador, 2014.

Hong, Euny. *The Power of Nunchi.* New York: Penguin Books, 2019.

Hong, Euny. "Watching South Korean TV Won't Make You Want to Have a Baby." *The New York Times*, June 19, 2025, http://nytimes.com/2025/06/19/opinion/k-drama-birthrate-crisis.html?campaign_id=39&emc=edit_ty_20250621&instance_id=156942&nl=opinion-today&regi_id=54871743&segment_id=200372&user_id=b445dde39e82461781cbfe0831ae61f9.

Hughes, Langston. "Theme for English B," accessed December 9, 2025, https://www.poetryfoundation.org/poems/47880/theme-for-english-b.

Hwang, Sok-yong. *The Guest*, translated by Kyung-Ja Chun and Maya West. New York: Seven Stories Press, 2006.

Ignatius, David. "Q&A: David Ignatius Answered Questions About His Spy Thriller, The Tao of Deception." *The Washington Post*, July 3, 2023, https://www.washingtonpost.com/opinions/2023/07/03/david-ignatius-ukraine-qa/.

Jamison, Kay Redfield. *Fires in the Dark: Healing the Unquiet Mind.* New York: Alfred A. Knopf, 2023.

Jenkins, Audrey Alyse. "Bedrock," in Maggie Azmitia, Megan Geers, Yeshi Mitiku, Audrey A. Jenkins, Natalie Briggs, Sasha Berger, Jackie Duncan, Bingjiefu He, and Mindy Fullilove, *One Step Can't Hurt: Situation Analysis Through the Lens of K-Drama*, pp. 24–36. New York: The New School, 2021.

Jirmanus, Lara Z., Rita M. Valenti, Eiryn A. Griest Schwartzman, Sophia A. Simon-Ortiz, Lauren I. Frey, Samuel R. Friedman, and Mindy T. Fullilove. "Too Many Deaths, Too Many Left Behind: A People's External Review of the US Centers for Disease Control and Prevention's COVID-19 Pandemic Response." *AJPM Focus* 3, no. 4 (2024): 100207.

Jung, Grace. *K-Drama School: A Pop Culture Inquiry into Why We Love Korean Television.* Philadelphia: Running Press, 2024.

Jung, Min-kyung. "Samppong: A Deep National Wound." *Korea Herald*, August 9, 2023. https://www.koreaherald.com/article/3188019.

Kim, Grace Ji-Sun. *Colonialism, Han, and the Transformative Spirit.* New York: Palgrave Macmillan, 2013.

Kim, Grace Ji-Sun. *The Homebrewed Christianity Guide to the Holy Spirit: Hand-Raisers, Han, and the Holy Ghost.* Minneapolis: Fortress Press, 2018.

Kim, Grace Ji-Sun. *When God Became White: Dismantling Whiteness for a More Just Christianity.* Downers Grove, IL: InterVarsity Press, 2024.

Kim, Halla. "Korean Philosophy (PDF Version)." *Stanford Encyclopedia of Philosophy*, 2022, https://plato.stanford.edu/entries/korean-philosophy/#:~:text=Korean%20philosophy%20is%20also%20characterized,are%20more%20primitive%20and%20real.

Kim, Kyung Hyun. *Hegemonic Mimicry: Korean Popular Culture of the Twenty-First Century.* Durham, NC: Duke University Press, 2021.

Kim, Kyung Hyun, and Youngmin Choe, eds. *The Korean Popular Culture Reader.* Durham, NC: Duke University Press, 2014.

Kimchi Mamas. "Oori," accessed May 26, 2025, https://kimchimamas.typepad.com/kimchi_mamas/2007/04/oori.html.

Kleinman, Arthur. *The Illness Narratives: Suffering, Healing, and the Human Condition.* New York: Basic Books, 1988.

Kleinman, Arthur. *Rethinking Psychiatry: From Cultural Category to Personal Experience.* New York: Free Press, 1991.

Kleinman, Arthur. *The Soul of Care: The Moral Education of a Husband and a Doctor.* New York: Viking, 2019.

Kleinman, Arthur. *What Really Matters: Living a Moral Life Amidst Uncertainty and Danger.* New York: Oxford University Press, 2006.

Kleinman, Arthur, Yunxiang Yan, Jing Jun, Sing Lee, Everett Zhang, Pan Tianshu, Wu Fei, and Jinhua Guo. *Deep China: The Moral Life of the Person.* Berkeley: University of California Press, 2011.

Ko, Kyung Soon. "A Broken Heart from a Wounded Land: The Use of a Korean Scarf Dance as a Dance/Movement Therapy Intervention for a Korean Woman with Haan." *The Arts in Psychotherapy* 55 (2017): 64–72. https://doi.org/10.1016/j.aip.2017.04.002.

Korea Clickers Facebook Page. "KOCIS of Ministry of Culture, Sports and Tourism, Jangheung Prison Aerial View," accessed July 2, 2024, https://www.facebook.com/photo/?fbid=378484617651730&set=pcb.378484744318384.

Korean History on a Page. "2014 Ferry Disaster Left Scars that Never Healed." *Korea Herald*, December 29, 2023, https://www.koreaherald.com/article/3290391.

The Korean. "The Forgotten Neoliberal Man of *Parasite*." *Ask a Korean*, accessed May 26, 2025, https://askakorean.blogspot.com/2020/03/the-forgotten-neoliberal-man-of-parasite.html?utm_source=dlvr.it&utm_medium=facebook.

Kraft, James. *The Works of Witter Bynner*. New York: Farrar, Straus, Giroux, 1978.

Kutcher, Norman. "The Fifth Relationship: Dangerous Friendships in the Confucian Context." *American Historical Review* 105, no. 5 (December 2000): 1615–1629.

Kuzmarov, Jeremy. "The Korean War: Barbarism Unleashed." US Foreign Policy History and Resource Guide website, 2016, https://peacehistory-usfp.org/korean-war.

Kwon, R. O. "Author R.O. Kwon's Guide to Seoul—Where She Loves to Eat, Drink, and Shop." *Travel + Leisure*, August 20, 2023, https://www.travelandleisure.com/seoul-korea-guide-with-r-o-kwon-7565463.

Laughter, Judson. "Toward a Theory of Micro-kindness: Developing Positive Actions in Multicultural Education." *International Journal of Multicultural Education* 16, no. 2 (2014): 2–14. https://doi.org/10.18251/ijme.v16i2.842.

Le Guin, Ursula K. *Lao Tzu Tao Te Ching: A Book About the Way and the Power of the Way*. Boulder, CO: Shambhala, 1997.

Lee, Jaeeun. "Two Years On, Thousands Mourn Itaewon Tragedy, Calling for Accountability." *Korea Times*, October 27, 2024, https://www.koreaherald.com/article/3832677.

Lieblich, Amia. *Seasons of Captivity: The Inner World of POWs*. New York: New York University Press, 1994.

Ling, L. M. H. *The Dao of World Politics: Towards a Post-Westphalian, Worldist International Relations*. New York: Routledge, 2014. https://doi.org/10.4324/9781315887777.

LollyPip. "Crash Landing on You: Episode 1." Dramabeans recaps, December 16, 2019, https://www.dramabeans.com/2019/12/crash-landing-on-you-episode-1/.

LollyPip, SailorJumun, and selena, "Crash Landing on You." Dramabeans recaps, 2019, accessed June 15, 2025, https://dramabeans.com/shows/crash-landing-on-you/.

Lucas, A. "The Date of the Exodus." *Palestine Exploration Quarterly* 73, no. 3 (1941): 110–121. https://doi.org/10.1179/peq.1941.73.3.110.

Lyrics Translate. "Happy End (English Ver.) Lyrics," accessed April 6, 2024, https://lyricstranslate.com/en/romance-bonus-book-ost-happy-end-english-ver-lyrics.html.

Lyrics Translate. "Happy End Lyrics," accessed April 6, 2024, https://lyricstranslate.com/en/romance-bonus-book-ost-happy-end-lyrics.html.

Lyrics Translate. "Hill of Yearning," accessed July 2, 2024, https://lyricstranslate.com/en/geulium-ui-eondeog-hill-yearning.html.

MacKinnon, Gillies, dir. *Regeneration*. 1997. Released in the US as *Behind the Lines*. Produced by Norstar Entertainment Inc. (Canada) and Rafford Films (UK).

Manker-Seale, Susan. “The Moral Arc of the Universe: Bending Toward Justice,” January 15, 2006, https://web.archive.org/web/20070811220256/http://www.uucnwt.org/sermons/TheMoralArcOfTheUniverse%201-15-06.html.

Maruyama, Ayako, Laura Van Vleet, Molly Rose Kaufman, Liam Van Vleet, and Mindy Thompson Fullilove. “The Laundry and the DMZ: Lessons for Trauma-Informed Placemaking,” in *Trauma Informed Placemaking*, edited by Cara Courage and Anita McKweon, pp. 36–44. London: Routledge, 2024.

Maryland Lynching Memorial. “Bryan Stevenson Quote,” accessed December 8, 2025, http://mdlynchingmemorial.org/.

Maté, Gabor. *When the Body Says No*. New York: Penguin Random House, 2019.

Matray, James I. “The Korean War 101: Causes, Course, and Conclusion of the Conflict.” *U.S., Asia, and the World: 1914–2012* 17, no. 3 (Winter 2012): 23–28. https://www.asianstudies.org/publications/eaa/archives/the-korean-war-101-causes-course-and-conclusion-of-the-conflict/.

Merriam-Webster Dictionary. “Athleisure Wear,” accessed July 2, 2024, https://www.merriam-webster.com/dictionary/athleisure#:~:text=%3A%20casual%20clothing%20designed%20to%20be,exercising%20and%20for%20general%20use.

Merriam-Webster.com Dictionary, s.v. “MacGyver,” accessed April 7, 2026, https://www.merriam-webster.com/dictionary/pragmatic.

Missvictrix and Sailor Jumun. “The King’s Affection: Episodes 1–20.” Dramabeans WeeCap, 2023, https://dramabeans.com/shows/the-kings-affection/.

Morales, Eduardo S., and Mindy Thompson Fullilove. “‘Many Are Called . . .’: Participation by Minority Leaders in an AIDS Intervention in San Francisco.” *Ethnicity & Disease* 21 (1992): 389–401.

Namu Wiki Editors:

“그냥 사랑하는 사이” (Just Between Lovers), last modified August 02, 2025, https://namu.wiki/w/어쩌다%20전원일기.

“나빌레라 (드라마)” (Navillera), last modified July 20, 2025, https://namu.wiki/w/나빌레라(드라마).

“낭만닥터 김사부” (Dr. Romantic), last modified July 09, 2025, https://namu.wiki/w/낭만닥터%20김사부.

“로맨스는 별책부록” (Romance Is a Bonus Book), last modified July 16, 2025, https://namu.wiki/w/로맨스는%20별책부록.

“명불허전(드라마)” (Live Up to Your Name), last modified August 05, 2025, https://namu.wiki/w/명불허전(드라마).

“미생(드라마)” (Misaeng: Incomplete Life), last modified August 05, 2025, https://namu.wiki/w/미생(드라마).

“사내맞선(드라마)” (Business Proposal), last modified August 05, 2025, https://namu.wiki/w/사내맞선(드라마).

“사랑의 불시착” (Crash Landing on You), last modified July 27, 2025, https://namu.wiki/w/사랑의%20불시착.

“세작, 매혹된 자들” (Captivating the King), last modified July 20, 2025, https://namu.wiki/w/세작%2C%20매혹된%20자들.

“슬기로운 감빵생활” (Prison Playbook), last modified August 04, 2025, https://namu.wiki/w/슬기로운%20감빵생활.

"어쩌다 전원일기" (Once Upon a Small Town), last modified July 15, 2025, https://namu.wiki/w/어쩌다%20전원일기.

"이상한 변호사 우영우" (Extraordinary Attorney Wu), last modified August 05, 2025, https://namu.wiki/w/이상한%20변호사%20우영우.

"더 킹: 영원의 군주" (The King: Eternal Monarch), last modified August 1, 2025, https://namu.wiki/w/더%20킹%20:%20영원의%20군주.

"연모" (The King's Affection), last modified July 20, 2025, https://namu.wiki/w/연모.

"웰컴투 삼달리" (Welcome to Samdal-ri), last modified July 20, 2025, https://namu.wiki/w/웰컴투%20삼달리.

"철인왕후(드라마)" (Mr. Queen), last modified August 03, 2025, https://namu.wiki/w/철인왕후(드라마).

Nazaryan, Alexander. "Bonds Beats the Babe! Statistical Model Crowns a New 'Greatest' in Baseball." *The New York Times*, August 12, 2025, https://www.nytimes.com/2025/08/12/science/baseball-statistics-babe-bonds.html.

Nelson, Scott Reynolds. "Steel Drivin' Man: John Henry, the Untold Story of an American Legend." *Virginia History*, accessed March 25, 2024, https://virginiahistory.org/learn/steel-drivin-man-john-henry-untold-story-american-legend#:~:text=According%20to%20the%20ballad%20that,beat%20the%20machine%2C%20and%20died.

OECD. "Health Status, Suicide Rates (Indicator)." *OECD iLibrary*, accessed April 8, 2024, https://doi.org/10.1787/a82f3459-en.

Owen, Wilfred. *Dulce et decorum est*. New York: Viking Press, 1921. Posted at The Poetry Foundation, accessed July 3, 2024, https://www.poetryfoundation.org/poems/46560/dulce-et-decorum-est.

Ó Tuama, Pádraig. *50 Poems to Open Your World*. New York: W. W. Norton & Company, 2022.

Polti, Georges. *The Thirty-Six Dramatic Situations*. Boston: The Writer, 1977.

Porter, Eleanor H. *Pollyanna*. Boston: The Page Company, 1913.

Prevost, Lisa. "Sylvia Ryerson's Calls from Home." *Yale News*, February 23, 2024, accessed May 26, 2025, https://news.yale.edu/2024/02/23/five-things-know-about-sylvia-ryersons-calls-home.

Prinz, Joachim. "Speech at the March on Washington," August 28, 1963, accessed August 16, 2025, https://www.americanjewisharchives.org/snapshots/the-problem-of-silence-rabbi-joachim-prinz-speech-at-the-march-on-washington/.

Puett, Michael, and Christine Gross-Loh. *The Path: What Chinese Philosophers Can Teach Us About the Good Life*. New York: Simon & Schuster, 2017.

quirkycase. "The King's Eternal Monarch: Episodes 1–16." Dramabeans recap, accessed June 15, 2025, https://dramabeans.com/shows/the-king-eternal-monarch/.

Quote Investigator. "There Are Only Two Plots: (1) A Person Goes on a Journey (2) A Stranger Comes to Town," May 6, 2015, accessed July 2, 2024. https://quoteinvestigator.com/2015/05/06/two-plots/.

Rennis, Lesley, Lourdes Hernández-Cordero, Kjersti Schmitz, and Mindy Thompson Fullilove. "'We Have a Situation Here!': Using Situation Analysis for Health and Social Research," in *Qualitative Research in Social Work*, edited by Anne E. Fortune, William J. Reid, and Robert Miller, pp. 192–212. New York: Columbia University Press, 2013.

Ringen, Stein, Huck-ju Kwon, Ilcheong Yi, Taekyoon Kim, and Jooha Lee. *The Korean State and Social Policy: How South Korea Lifted Itself from Poverty and Dictatorship to Affluence and Democracy*. New York: Oxford University Press, 2011.

Rivers, W. H. R. *Conflict and Dream*. New York: Routledge, 2014.

Rivers, W. H. R. *Instinct and the Unconscious: A Contribution to a Biological Theory of the Psycho-Neurosis*, 2nd ed. Cambridge: Cambridge University Press, 2014.

Rohr, Richard. "Possessed by the Wrong Perspective." Richard Rohr's Daily Meditations from the Center for Action and Contemplation, January 27, 2025, https://email.cac.org/t/d-e-sjjuho-tyltukthjy-w/.

Rosman, Katherine. "He Was One of the Central Park Five. Now He's Councilman Yusef Salaam." *The New York Times*, December 31, 2023, https://www.nytimes.com/2023/12/31/nyregion/yusef-salaam-central-park-five-city-council.html.

RWJBarnabas Health. "Why Trauma Matters: A New Model of Compassionate Care Recognized How Past Events Can Affect Health and Behavior." *Healthy Together*, Summer 2024, pp. 6–7.

SailorJumun. "The King's Affection: Episodes 19-20 Open Thread (Final)." Dramabeans recaps, December 16, 2021, https://www.dramabeans.com/2021/12/the-kings-affection-episodes-19-20-open-thread-final/comment-page-3/.

Salesses, Matthew. *Craft in the Real World*. New York: Catapult, 2021.

Sassoon, Siegfried. *Sherston's Progress: The Memoirs of George Sherston*. New York: Penguin Books, 1964.

Sassoon, Siegfried. "To a Very Wise Man," quoted in Kay Redfield Jamison, *Fires in the Dark: Healing the Mind, the Oldest Branch of Medicine*, p. 97. New York: Alfred A. Knopf, 2023.

Schmitt, Major John F., and Gary A. Klein. "Fighting in the Fog: Dealing with Battlefield Uncertainty." *Marine Corps Gazette* 80, no. 8 (August 1996): 69.

Shakespeare, William. "Midsummer Night's Dream." Folger Shakespeare Library, accessed July 2, 2024, https://www.folger.edu/explore/shakespeares-works/a-midsummer-nights-dream/read/.

Shakespeare, William. "The Complete Works of William Shakespeare, Life and Death of Julius Caesar." William Shakespeare, Julius Caesar (Act 4, Scene 3), spoken by Brutus, accessed April 7, 2026, https://shakespeare.mit.edu/julius_caesar/julius_caesar.4.3.html.

Shankman, Sabrina. "Cumberland Divided: Maine Governor Mills's Stand Against Trump Splits a Small Town." *Boston Globe*, February 24, 2025, https://www.bostonglobe.com/2025/02/24/metro/maine-governor-mills-transgender-trump/?et_rid=50004187&s_campaign=todaysheadlines:newsletter.

Situation Analysis Through the Lens of K-Drama Fall 2021 Class. *One Step Can't Hurt: Situation Analysis Through the Lens of K-Drama*. Report of Analysis of the K-Drama "Crash Landing on You," The New School, Fall 2021.

Situation Analysis Through the Lens of K-Drama Spring 2024 Class. *Tides of Hope: Situation Analysis Through the Lens of K-Drama*. Report of Analysis of the K-Drama "Our Blues," The New School, 2024.

Small, Deborah. "Introduction," in Kang Han, *Human Acts*, pp. 1–5. London: Granta Books, 2020.

Smiles, Herbert. "Hope Is Like the Sun," quoted in LaNysha T. Adams, "The 3-31 from Dr. Adams," May 4, 2022, accessed July 2, 2024, https://www.ourmepower.com/p/hope-is-like-the-sun.

Spotify. "Powerdance," accessed May 26, 2025, https://open.spotify.com/track/2Z6nTtGATaLpoldT9LXAl3.

Stack, Liam. "Korean War, a 'Forgotten' Conflict That Shaped the Modern World." *The New York Times*, January 1, 2018, https://www.nytimes.com/2018/01/01/world/asia/korean-war-history.htm.

Stone, I. F. *The Hidden History of the Korean War*. New York: Monthly Review Press, 1952.

Sullivan, Robert. "The Town Shrink." *New York Times Magazine*, June 23, 2015, https://www.nytimes.com/2015/06/28/magazine/the-town-shrink.html.

Sunny and abirdword. "Romance Is a Bonus Book." Dramabeans recaps, 2023, accessed June 15, 2025, https://dramabeans.com/shows/romance-is-a-bonus-book/.

Tatar, Maria. *The Grimm Reader: The Classic Tales of the Brothers Grimm*. New York: W. W. Norton, 2010.

Tatar, Maria. *The Heroine with 1001 Faces*. New York: Liveright Publishing, 2021.

Thompson, Ernest, and Mindy Thompson. *Homebody Came to Orange: A Story of People's Power*. Orange, NJ: Bridgebuilder Press, 1976 (reissued, New York: New Village Press, 2018).

Thompson, Mindy. *The National Negro Labor Council: A History, 1951–1956*. Senior Honors Thesis, Bryn Mawr College, 1971.

Tse-Tung, Mao. *On Contradiction*, 1937, accessed May 26, 2025, https://www.marxists.org/reference/archive/mao/selected-works/volume-1/mswv1_17.htm.

Tudor, Daniel. *Korea: The Impossible Country*. North Clarendon, VT: Tuttle Publishing, 2018.

Twain, Mark. "Father," accessed March 31, 2024, http://www.twainquotes.com/Father.html.

Vadukul, Alex. "The Unlikely Friendship That Saved a Dive Bar." *The New York Times*, March 18, 2025, https://www.nytimes.com/2025/03/18/style/lucys-ny-bar-renovation.html?campaign_id=61&emc=edit_ts_20250318&instance_id=150322&nl=the-great-read&regi_id=54871743&segment_id=193774&user_id=b445dde39e82461781cbfe0831ae61f9.

van der Kolk, Bessel A. *The Body Keeps the Score*. New York: Penguin Books, 2014.

van der Kolk, Bessel A., Nan Herron, and Ann Hostetler. "The History of Trauma in Psychiatry." *Psychiatric Clinics of North America* 17, no. 3 (1994): 583–600.

VarietyRecaps. "Just Between Lovers Recaps, Episodes 1–16," accessed July 1, 2024, https://varietyrecaps.wordpress.com/2018/01/06/just-between-lovers-ep-2/.

Visit Korea. "Seodaemun Prison History Museum (서대문형무소역사관)," accessed April 7, 2024, https://english.visitkorea.or.kr/svc/whereToGo/locIntrdn/locIntrdnList.do?vcontsId=111259&menuSn=351.

Wallace, Anthony F. C. "Mazeway Disintegration: The Individual's Perception of Socio-Cultural Disorganization." *Human Organization* 16, no. 2 (Summer 1957): 23–27.

Wallace, Rodrick. *Carl von Clausewitz, the Fog-of-War, and the AI Revolution: The Real World Is Not a Game of Go*. Cham, Switzerland: Springer, 2018.

Wallace, Rodrick. "Fog, Friction, and Failure in Organized Conflict: A Formal Study." *Axioms* 13, no. 2 (2024): 111. https://doi.org/10.3390/axioms13020111.

Wallace, Rodrick, and Mindy Thompson Fullilove. *Collective Consciousness and Its Discontents: Institutional Distributed Cognition, Racial Policy and Public Health in the United States*. New York: Springer Science & Business Media, 2007.

Wallace, Rodrick, Deborah Wallace, J. E. Ullmann, and Howard Andrews. "Deindustrialization, Inner-City Decay, and the Hierarchical Diffusion of AIDS in the USA: How Neoliberal and Cold War Policies Magnified the Ecological Niche for Emerging Infections and Created a National Security Crisis." *Environment and Planning A* 31, no. 1 (January 1999): 113–139.

War and Women's Human Rights Museum. "About Us," accessed April 6, 2024, https://womenandwarmuseum.net/updates-eng.

Watkins, Beverly X., Robert E. Fullilove, and Mindy Thompson Fullilove. "Arms Against Illness: Crack Cocaine and US Drug Policy." *Health and Human Rights* 2 (1998): 43–58.

Wells, Catharine P. "Microaggressions: What They Are and Why They Matter." *Texas Hispanic Journal of Law and Policy* 24, no. 1 (September 2017): 61–80.

Wikipedia Editors:

"Aging of South Korea," last modified March 29, 2024, https://en.wikipedia.org/wiki/Aging_of_South_Korea.

"Because This Is My First Life," last modified June 29, 2025, https://en.wikipedia.org/wiki/Because_This_Is_My_First_Life.

"Business Proposal," last modified July 25, 2025, https://en.wikipedia.org/wiki/Business_Proposal.

"Captivating the King," last modified April 8, 2025, https://en.wikipedia.org/wiki/Captivating_the_King

"Central Park Jogger Case," last modified July 1, 2024, https://en.wikipedia.org/wiki/Central_Park_jogger_case.

"Crash Landing on You," last modified June 8, 2025, https://en.wikipedia.org/wiki/Crash_Landing_on_You.

"Dr. Romantic," last modified July 25, 2025, https://en.wikipedia.org/wiki/Dr._Romantic.

"Extraordinary Attorney Wu," last modified July 26, 2025, https://en.wikipedia.org/wiki/Extraordinary_Attorney_Woo.

"Fog of War," last modified March 19, 2024, https://en.wikipedia.org/wiki/Fog_of_war.

"Heo Im," last modified March 25, 2024, https://en.wikipedia.org/wiki/Heo_Im.

"Heo Jun," last modified June 14, 2025, https://en.wikipedia.org/wiki/Heo_Jun.

"Hospital Volunteers," last modified March 9, 2025, https://en.wikipedia.org/wiki/Hospital_volunteer.

"Just Between Lovers/Rain or Shine," last modified April 29, 2025, https://en.wikipedia.org/wiki/Rain_or_Shine_(TV_series).

"The King: Eternal Monarch," last modified May 12, 2025, https://en.wikipedia.org/wiki/The_King:_Eternal_Monarch.

"The King's Affection," last modified February 25, 2025, https://en.wikipedia.org/wiki/The_King%27s_Affection.

"Live Up to Your Name," last modified April 10, 2025, https://en.wikipedia.org/wiki/Live_Up_to_Your_Name.

"Misaeng: Incomplete Life," last modified July 25, 2025, https://en.wikipedia.org/wiki/:_Incomplete_Life.

"Mr. Queen Controversies," last modified February 25, 2025, https://en.wikipedia.org/wiki/Mr._Queen#Controversies.

"My Liberation Notes," last modified July 26, 2025, https://en.wikipedia.org/wiki/My_Liberation_Notes.

"Navillera," last modified July 10, 2025, https://en.wikipedia.org/wiki/Navillera_(TV_series).

"Once Upon a Small Town," last modified August 7, 2025, https://en.wikipedia.org/wiki/Once_Upon_a_Small_Town.

"Poong, the Joseon Psychiatrist," last modified July 12, 2025, https://en.wikipedia.org/wiki/Poong,_the_Joseon_Psychiatrist.

"Prison Playbook," last modified May 15, 2025, https://en.wikipedia.org/wiki/Prison_Playbook.

"Romance Is a Bonus Book," last modified April 8, 2025, https://en.wikipedia.org/wiki/Romance_Is_a_Bonus_Book.

"Veritable Records of the Joseon Dynasty," last modified June 9, 2025, https://en.wikipedia.org/wiki/Veritable_Records_of_the_Joseon_Dynasty.

"Welcome to Samdal-ri," last updated July 16, 2025, https://en.wikipedia.org/wiki/Welcome_to_Samdal-ri.

Wilson, Jean Moorcroft. "Dr W. H.R. Rivers: Siegfried Sassoon and Robert Graves' 'fathering friend.'" *Brain* 140 (2017): 3378–3383.

Yasir, Sameer. "Where 'No One Wanted Girls,' a Dad in India Takes On the Patriarchy." *The New York Times*, August 4, 2023, https://www.nytimes.com/2023/08/04/world/asia/sunil-jaglan-india-haryana-womens-rights.html?campaign_id=61&emc=edit_ts_20230804&instance_id=99251&nl=the-great-read&regi_id=54871743&segment_id=141140&te=1&user_id=b445dde39e82461781cbfe0831ae61f9.

Yoon, L. "Suicide in South Korea: Statistics and Facts." *Statista*, February 2, 2024, https://www.statista.com/topics/8622/suicide-in-south-korea/#:~:text=South%20Korea%20has%20the%20highest,their%20own%20lives%20in%202021.

Zauner, Michelle. *Crying in H-Mart: A Memoir*. New York: Alfred A. Knopf, 2022.

Zuckerman, Esther. "Are We in a New Golden Age for the Movie Soundtrack?" *The New York Times*, May 17, 2025, https://www.nytimes.com/2024/05/17/movies/barbie-spider-verse-i-saw-the-tv-glow-soundtrack.html.

Index

For the benefit of digital users, indexed terms that span two pages (e.g., 52–53) may, on occasion, appear on only one of those pages.